THE EPILEPSY REFERENCE BOOK

Dr Jolyon Oxley, MA, MB, BCHIR, MRCP is well known nationally and internationally for his work in epilepsy. He was Medical Director of the National Society for Epilepsy for ten years. During that time he developed a particular interest in the drug treatment and the social aspects of epilepsy, and is currently chairman of the Commission on Employment of the International Bureau for Epilepsy. He is also chairman of the external advisory group on rehabilitation for the National Society for Epilepsy. In the last two years he has pursued an interest in medical education, and is currently Secretary of the Standing Committee on Postgraduate Medical Education. He lives in London.

Dr Jay Smith, MBBS, FRANZCP trained as a psychiatrist in Australia before moving to the UK. She has an interest in long-term illness, and currently works part-time on a psychiatric rehabilitation unit. She also works as a freelance journalist, specializing in medical educational material. She lives in London.

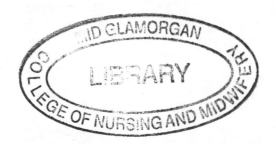

The Epilepsy Reference Book

Jolyon Oxley *and* Jay Smith

First published in 1991
by Faber and Faber Ltd
3 Queen Square London WC1N 3AU

Photoset by Parker Typesetting Service, Leicester
Printed in England by Clays Ltd, St Ives plc

© Jolyon Oxley and Jay Smith, 1991

Jolyon Oxley and Jay Smith are hereby identified as authors of this work in
accordance with Section 77 of the Copyright, Designs and Patents Act 1988

The first edition of this book was written by Professor Peter Jeavons and
Alec Aspinall of the British Epilepsy Association.

A CIP record for this book is available from the British Library.

ISBN 0 571 16253 3

Contents

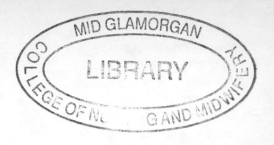

Illustrations

Acknowledgments

We have been helped by many people with experience of epilepsy who have read the manuscript, offered comments and suggested questions. The contributions of people with epilepsy and their relatives have been especially valuable. In addition, people who work in the field of epilepsy in one way or another have given us the benefit of their advice, especially Vivienne Cairnie, Epilepsy Association of Scotland; Brian Chappell, British Epilepsy Association; David Eking, National Society for Epilepsy; Barbara Hawkins, West London Action for Epilepsy Group; Maggie Heaton, British Epilepsy Association; Richard Holmes, Irish Epilepsy Association; Carole Rossington, Croydon Epilepsy Society. We would also like to thank Jane Archibald, Jean Clarke, Irving and Ann Elmer, Ingrid Gibson, Cynthia Green, Jenny Hallow, Clifford Hanley, Ken Hewson, Eileen Holloway, Judith Lanfear, Susan Lannon, Maurice Parsonage, Michael Roberts, Elizabeth Simmers, Roger Symes, Sue Usiskin and Mark Williams.

1 How to use this book

Although epilepsy is common throughout the world, people with
epilepsy still come across a lot of ignorance about their condition.
Information about epilepsy is the key to fighting prejudice in daily life
and making sure that all people with epilepsy receive the best possible
treatment and are able to enjoy life to the full. As is stated in the
British Epilepsy Association's Charter (see page 141), people with
epilepsy 'deserve quality medical care from practitioners who understand epilepsy ... [and] have the right to information to help them
choose whether or not to undergo any treatment offered'. And as
William McLin of the Epilepsy Federation of America added recently,
'Well-informed patients make sure their doctors are well-informed.'

How this book is organized

This book has been designed to inform you about epilepsy in its
broadest sense – what the condition is, how it is treated, what it feels
like to have epilepsy and what it is like to live with. It is written in a
question-and-answer format and the questions are based on those
most commonly asked by people with epilepsy and their families. In
formulating the questions we have relied on advice from people with
epilepsy as well as professionals working in the field. Because
everyone's experience of epilepsy is different, we have answered
questions asked by a range of different people – those with epilepsy
themselves, and their friends and relatives, including mothers and
fathers of children with epilepsy.

The chapters have been organized to answer the most immediate questions before looking at other issues. So Chapters 2 and 3 give an overview of the diagnosis of epilepsy and how developing epilepsy may affect a person's life. The next important issue is treatment, which is dealt with in Chapter 4. In Chapter 5 we look at questions about the different seizure types and other basic information about patterns of epilepsy. Chapter 6 examines the drugs in more detail. Chapters 7 and 8 are concerned with questions which arise in two different situations: when seizures stop, and when they don't. The many aspects of living with epilepsy are discussed in Chapter 9. Chapter 10 looks at epilepsy in the future and what can be done to help now. You will find useful addresses listed at the end of the book, and also on pages 112 and 126.

Using this book

One of the difficulties of writing about epilepsy is that it affects so many different people. The questions which the parents of a three-year-old boy with epilepsy might ask are very different from those which will concern a twenty-five year-old woman. Another difficulty is that epilepsy varies so much in its nature and severity that each person's experience of the condition is unique in some way. We have tried to look at all angles and to organize the questions in a logical way. However, you may well find that some questions in every chapter are helpful to you, while others are not relevant. Even if your seizures are well controlled, you may find some interesting information in Chapter 7, which we have called 'My fits haven't stopped yet'. We expect that everyone will use the book in a different way. To help you decide which parts might be important to you, we have included a brief introduction at the beginning and a summary at the end of each chapter.

As you read this book, you may notice that we often recommend seeking counselling or advice. Unfortunately, this is not always as easy to find as it should be – but it is worth persevering until you find

what you need. We have supplied contact names and addresses to
help you in your search.

A word about names

The terms used in epilepsy can be quite confusing. In the questions
and answers, we have used the words 'seizure', 'fit' and 'attack', as
these words are all in common use to describe the same thing.
Medical names for the different seizures are explained in the book,
but we have included brief explanations of some of the most common terms here.

Useful terms

Absence seizure: a brief seizure, usually in children, where the
person 'loses touch' for a few seconds but does not fall.

Anti-convulsant: a rather old-fashioned term for a drug which is
used to treat epilepsy.

Anti-epileptic: a general name for a group of drugs which are used
in the treatment of epilepsy.

Atonic seizure: a type of seizure where the person suddenly
becomes limp and falls forward.

Aura: a warning of a seizure, which may take a number of forms
such as a feeling in the stomach or a strange smell.

Clonic seizure: a seizure during which rapid, jerking, to-and-fro
movements of the arms and legs occur.

Complex partial seizure: a seizure which involves part of the
brain ('partial') and there is some loss of contact with the outside
world ('complex'). The events which occur in a partial seizure
depend on which part of the brain is affected.

Convulsion: an old-fashioned term for a tonic-clonic seizure (see
below).

CT scan: a special x-ray which gives a detailed image of the
structure of the brain.

EEG: a painless test which records electrical patterns in the brain. These may show signs of seizures.

Epilepsy: a tendency to recurrent seizures due to a brain disorder.

Generalized seizures: seizures which involve the whole of the brain from the beginning. There are six types of generalized seizure (absence, myoclonic, tonic-clonic, tonic, clonic and atonic).

Myoclonic seizures: sudden jerks of the muscles in the arms, legs or body, which may be repeated.

Partial seizures: seizures which involve a part of the brain.

Seizure: A sudden electrical discharge of brain cells, resulting in movement of the body or changes in behaviour.

Serum level monitoring: this term refers to blood tests which reveal the amount of a drug present in the blood (and thus in other parts of the body).

Simple partial seizure: a seizure involving one part of the brain. The person remains in touch with the world and aware of what is happening.

Tonic seizure: a seizure where stiffening of the body occurs and the person falls over.

Tonic-clonic seizure: in this type of seizure, the person goes stiff, falls to the ground and then has jerking movements of the body.

2 I've just been told I've got epilepsy

This chapter takes you through the process of diagnosis. Experiencing fits and then hearing the diagnosis of epilepsy are big events in anyone's life. We look at the sort of information that doctors need, and explain how tests can help doctors reach a decision. We then explore some of the issues involved in coming to terms with the diagnosis. Often people are too shocked and bewildered to remember much of what their doctors say at this stage.

. . . .

How do doctors know that I've got epilepsy?
Epilepsy is an unusual condition because you can't see it and you can't do a test to prove that it's there. Epilepsy is a disorder of the brain that only shows itself when the person affected has a fit or seizure. As these don't occur very often, for most of the time the person's brain is working entirely normally.

So to make a diagnosis doctors have to rely entirely on knowing in detail what has actually happened to you both in the course of your everyday life and at the time when you had the unusual experience that was thought to have been a fit. This part of the diagnostic process is called 'the history' and is absolutely crucial to everything that happens later.

What information did the doctor use to make a diagnosis?
Both you and the people who have seen your attacks will have given vital information. You were probably asked a lot of questions and

generally these had three aims. First of all, the doctor needed to decide whether what happened to you was a seizure or not. At the same time, the doctor asked about things which might help to decide what kind of seizure you had. Lastly, the doctor tried to establish if there was an obvious reason for your having had a fit.

The kinds of question generally asked about the event itself are shown in the following list.

Questions your doctor may ask to make a diagnosis

1 Before the event

What were you doing at the time?
Did you feel strange in any way or have any sort of warning?
Did you seem moody or different?
Had anything unusual happened (for example, a late night, a party with a lot of drinking?)
Had you had any sort of emotional upset just before?
Had you had a meal recently?
Had you taken any kind of drug?
What time of day was it?

2 During the event

What did you feel?
What was the first thing that anyone noticed happening to you?
What happened to your body and where did the seizure start?
In what order did events happen – for example, did your head turn, followed by movements of the face and then movements of the arms and legs?
Did you fall and, if so, how?
Did your body become stiff?
Was there jerking and twitching, and if so, where?
Did you black out or seem out of touch with your surroundings?
Did your breathing change?

Did your face change colour?
Did you pass water during the event?
Were there any injuries?

3 After the event

How long was it until you were back to normal?
Did you recover quickly or gradually?
Were you drowsy?
Did you complain of a headache or were you sick?
Did you do anything odd afterwards, like wandering around?

As well as all this information, your doctor will want to know details of any other illnesses or injuries that you have had, going right back to your childhood. So it's as well to ask your mother or father about this, if possible, before you visit the specialist. You will also be asked whether you have ever experienced fits before, including those sometimes called 'teething fits' or febrile convulsions (see page 43). Finally, the doctor will need to know about other members of your family and whether any of them have had a similar problem. In some families the word 'fit' may not be used, 'turn', 'funny do' or 'blackout' being used instead.

What exactly happens when I have a fit?

In the brain, cells communicate with each other all the time. This is illustrated in the diagram on page 8. The flow of information from cell to cell is very precisely controlled. A seizure occurs when brain transmission begins to malfunction, sending rapid and uncontrolled messages. This disorganized and excessive activity usually only lasts for a few seconds or minutes. But it may cause disturbances of sensation, movement or alertness, depending on which area of the brain is involved.

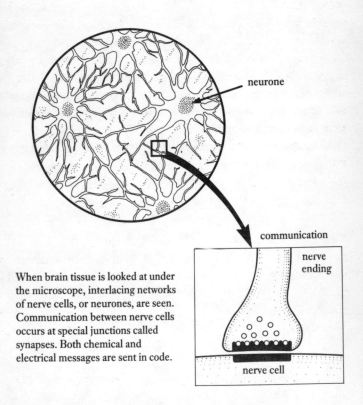

neurone

communication

nerve
ending

When brain tissue is looked at under
the microscope, interlacing networks
of nerve cells, or neurones, are seen.
Communication between nerve cells
occurs at special junctions called
synapses. Both chemical and
electrical messages are sent in code.

nerve cell

Communication in the brain

After my first fit, nobody told me that I had epilepsy. Why are they saying this now?

A lot of people (about one in twenty) have a single fit at some point in their lives. We don't know exactly how many people go on to have more attacks. Research work from the UK suggests that as many as six out of ten people, having had one fit, will have another within twelve months. Other work from the USA suggests that this number is rather smaller, about three or four out of ten. So after a first fit we can't be sure whether there will be any more or not. Sometimes there are features in a person's past history, a really bad injury to the head, for example, that would suggest that he or she is likely to have more attacks. But often this isn't the case, so we wait and see what happens. If more fits occur, then a diagnosis of epilepsy is usually made.

Although it's rather complicated, a definition of epilepsy may help at this stage:

> Epilepsy can be defined as 'a persistent tendency to fits or seizures which occur as a result of a brain disorder'.

What is the difference between a fit and a seizure?

None. In the UK the word 'fit' is used widely although it is associated in most people's minds with a convulsion (or grand mal fit, see page 47) and not with other types of attack. 'Seizure' is the preferred term in the USA and is catching on in the UK too. Sometimes other terms are used, such as 'attack', 'turn' or 'spell', which are perhaps less alarming. Even the word 'epilepsy' is not liked by some, who prefer the term 'seizure disorder'. Whatever words you use it is important to make sure that you and your advisors understand exactly what you all mean. Wherever possible, the international classification should be used as the various terms have precise meanings. A summary of the international classification is shown on page 10 and is discussed in further detail in Chapter 5.

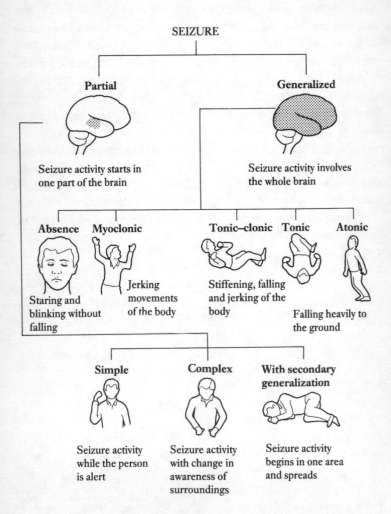

SEIZURE

Partial

Seizure activity starts in one part of the brain

Generalized

Seizure activity involves the whole brain

Absence

Staring and blinking without falling

Myoclonic

Jerking movements of the body

Tonic–clonic

Stiffening, falling and jerking of the body

Tonic

Atonic

Falling heavily to the ground

Simple

Seizure activity while the person is alert

Complex

Seizure activity with change in awareness of surroundings

With secondary generalization

Seizure activity begins in one area and spreads

Classification of seizures

How do you know that this tendency to have fits will persist in my case?
Sometimes there is evidence that a person's brain is permanently
damaged and thereby made more susceptible to fits indefinitely, but
often we can't be sure what will happen in the future. Research
studies in the UK have shown that six out of ten people having had
one fit will have another one within twelve months. Once a second
fit has occurred, the chances of more are even higher.

*The definition of epilepsy mentions fits due to a brain disorder. What is
meant by 'a disorder'?*
Most of the illnesses that we all get are due to viruses or bacteria.
We are well; then the virus or bacteria comes along and we fall ill
with various symptoms. The body gets rid of the virus or bacteria
and we recover. Other ailments, for example arthritis, may be due to
the body wearing out as we get older. Epilepsy isn't like either of
these types of illness. In many people we think that epilepsy is due
to some in-built property within the brain which prevents it from
controlling its own activity properly, and this failure results in fits.

In many cases we can only speculate about the cause. In the
instance just described it is probably due to a chemical imbalance
within the person's brain which leads to the brain's messages
suddenly becoming disorganized. In other cases, however, the
cause is more obvious. The person affected may have suffered an
injury to the head or a stroke which has damaged the brain. This
damage stops the brain controlling its activity and makes the person
susceptible to fits.

Is it right to call epilepsy a disease?
Epilepsy is not usually thought of as a disease. This term tends to
mean something which is likely to progress and could involve
several areas of the body. Epilepsy involves a temporary disturbance
in the function of the brain.

Can fits occur for other reasons?

Yes, they can, but they are uncommon. Perhaps the commonest cause of fits, other than epilepsy, is too much alcohol which can lead to 'blackouts', in fact a form of fit. Rarely, people with diabetes can have a fit if their blood sugar falls too low, either because of lack of food or too much insulin. Other types of illness which produce severe abnormalities in the body's chemistry (for example, kidney failure) can also cause fits. But in comparison to epilepsy, these are rare causes.

Older people may start having fits because of damage to the brain such as can occur in a stroke (see page 133). The one thing that many people fear is a brain tumour. Tumours are very uncommon in children and young people but should be looked for in adults who start having fits for the first time.

Special tests

Why did my doctor do blood tests?

Blood tests are useful in trying to detect any underlying disease which may be causing the fits. They can give information about the functioning of the liver and kidneys, and the state of the blood. In addition, blood tests for vitamin deficiency, or to find toxins in the body, may be ordered if your medical history and physical examination suggest that these factors may be involved.

Blood tests are also used as 'base line' information, because anti-epileptic drugs can occasionally affect various aspects of body functioning (see Chapter 4). So most doctors like to have an idea of these functions before they prescribe anti-epileptic drugs.

What is an EEG?

The EEG, which is a short way of saying electroencephalogram, is a test which records the electrical activity occurring inside the brain. Electrical activity is a central part of the communication between brain cells, and seizures occur when there is abnormal electrical discharge of these cells. In the late 1920s it was discovered that electrical signals from the brain could be recorded by electrodes placed on the scalp. In epilepsy (and other brain conditions) these electrical patterns may show changes which can help make the diagnosis. Two examples of EEG tracings are shown in the diagram below.

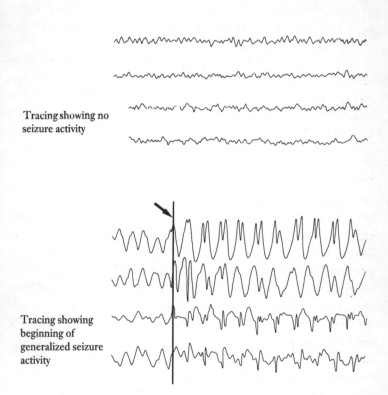

Tracing showing no
seizure activity

Tracing showing
beginning of
generalized seizure
activity

Two examples of EEG tracings

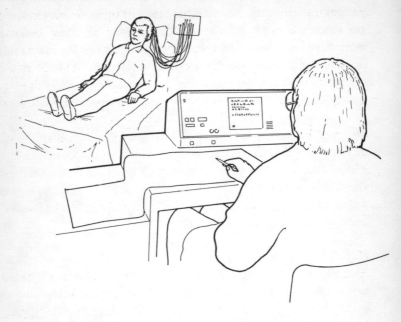

Recording an EEG

I have to have an EEG. What will happen?
The EEG is a simple, painless test. Pads (or electrodes) are placed on the head, and may be stuck to your scalp with a special glue. In the routine EEG, up to twenty electrodes are placed in standard positions on the head. The electrical impulses picked up by the pads are conducted by wires into the EEG machine, where they are amplified 100,000 times and printed out on to paper. The recording usually takes about thirty minutes; during this time you will be asked to lie quite still, as contraction of muscles can show up on the EEG, making interpretation difficult.

The main complaint from people after an EEG is having to wash the glue out of their hair, so don't have your hair done before you go for the test!

Will I have to do anything during the test?
Various methods may be used during the recording in order to see if any abnormalities are present. For example, the EEG may become more clearly abnormal when the person breathes rapidly, so you will be asked to breathe quickly for several minutes. This is called overbreathing or *hyperventilation*. Similarly, some abnormalities show up better during sleep, so you may be allowed to doze off during the test.

My friend said flashing lights were used during the EEG test. Why is that?
In some people, flashing lights bring on abnormal activity on the EEG. This is called photosensitivity, a relatively rare condition which is always tested for when recording an EEG. If present, you will be advised to avoid certain patterns of flashing light which could make you have a seizure.

Why do I need to have an EEG?
An EEG will give your doctor a lot of useful information. First, it may help support the diagnosis of epilepsy. Second, it may also be used to decide what type of seizure you are having. The role of triggering factors (such as flashing lights or overbreathing) may also be shown.

My EEG is normal. Does that mean I don't have epilepsy?
Many people with epilepsy have a normal EEG in between seizures, so that a normal EEG does not mean you do not have epilepsy. A surprising number of people who have never had seizures show 'epileptic patterns' on their EEG. So the EEG is used to support other information which your doctor will use to make a diagnosis. The diagnosis of epilepsy is never made on the EEG alone.

What is a CT scan?
Technically, it is a series of special x-rays which picture the brain in 'slices'. When these slices are viewed in order, the doctor is able to build up a picture of the whole brain.
    The CT scan, also known as a CAT scan or computerized axial

tomography, may provide very helpful information about the structure of the brain, in contrast to the information about function
provided by the EEG. A CT scan may help to reveal the cause of the
epilepsy but does not tell whether or not the person has epilepsy in
the first place.

Do I need a scan?
This is a decision which will be made by your doctor, who has all the
information about your condition. A CT scan is not necessary for
every person who has seizures, and is only normally advised if the
doctor suspects there may be something wrong with the structure of
the brain which is causing the fits. A CT scan is more commonly
used if a person has a seizure for the first time in adult life, when
doctors may be worried that the person has a brain tumour.

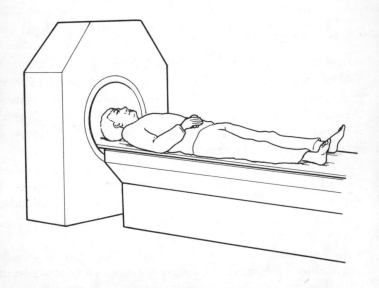

Having a CT scan

Are CT scans painful?
No. The person lies down while the machine takes a series of x-ray pictures. The diagram opposite shows you what it is like to have one. Occasionally an injection into an arm vein is given of a 'contrast material' which helps to show up parts of the brain.

When my baby son had a convulsion, the doctor at the hospital did a lumbar puncture. Why was this done?
In a lumbar puncture some of the fluid surrounding the brain is drained through a needle put into the person's back at the base of the spine. It's not a very pleasant thing to have done but shouldn't be too painful, if performed expertly. The fluid can be examined for signs of infection such as meningitis.

This test is not used routinely, but is only done if the circumstances of the seizure indicate an infection.

Questioning the diagnosis

So how can you really be sure that I've got epilepsy?
Doctors cannot be 100 per cent positive unless they've actually seen you have a number of attacks or received reliable eye-witness accounts of your repeated attacks. They also need to exclude all other possible causes for the fits. The way that the diagnosis is reached is summarized in the diagram on page 8.

Most doctors do not see their patients having attacks and so accurate information from you and reliable eye-witnesses is absolutely crucial to getting the diagnosis right. It is very helpful to have a written description of the seizures with the answers to the kinds of question listed earlier in this chapter.

Unfortunately in a few cases these reliable accounts are missing and yet the diagnosis is still made. Epilepsy can be quite easily mistaken for a number of other conditions. Once the diagnosis is made it is very difficult to change it, particularly if treatment has been started. Doctors tend to be cautious about changing the

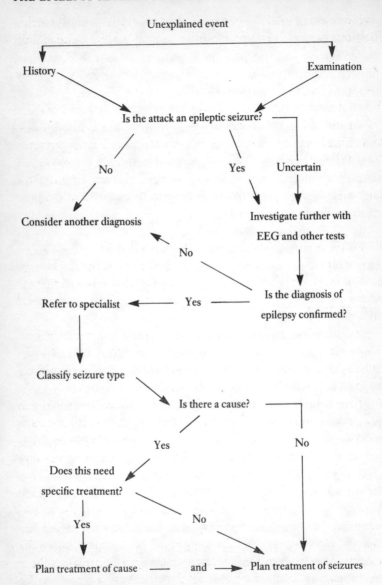

Diagnosing epilepsy

diagnosis which will have been made by a colleague. Unfortunately a diagnosis can tend to become 'written in stone' so that no one thinks to question it.

Can my GP make the diagnosis alone?
Yes, but most won't. Your GP is in a key position to record detailed information about the attacks as soon after the events as possible. It is surprising how much important information can be forgotten later. Your GP will also know a lot about your medical history and family details and can pass this on to the hospital consultant. But it is the hospital consultant who usually arranges tests and who will tell you about the diagnosis.

Should the diagnosis be reviewed and who should do this?
The best person to review the diagnosis with you is the doctor who made it in the first place. If this is not possible then it is vital that the doctor carrying out the review has access to all the background information.

How often the diagnosis should be reviewed is a more difficult matter. If you continue to have fits, however infrequently, the epilepsy clearly hasn't gone away. Even if the attacks appear to have stopped, we cannot be entirely sure that they won't return.

There is another complicating factor. Most people are advised to take drug treatment after their second fit. If no more occur, we cannot know whether the epilepsy has gone away or whether it is just the drugs that are controlling the fits. This uncertainty can be very frustrating.

It is normal practice to wait for at least two years after the last fit has occurred before trying to stop treatment. If the drugs are stopped successfully and no further attacks occur over the next one to two years then it is reasonable to say that the person no longer has epilepsy. If during or after the withdrawal of treatment, more fits happen, then obviously the problem is still there. Unfortunately there is no other way to find out for sure if the epilepsy is still present. An EEG may be helpful sometimes.

I don't want to accept the diagnosis of epilepsy. What can I do?
There are two aspects to this question. The simpler one concerns making sure the diagnosis is right. You can always ask for another opinion. But before doing so, it's sensible to talk over your concern and find out if the doctor is also uncertain and if more information would help. If you do decide to consult another doctor, it's very important that the doctor has all the information, including eye-witness accounts. All the results of tests need to be available. It's also important that the doctor you consult is the right one. Not all doctors, even specialists, have the same level of expertise in all areas. The best people to advise you about getting another opinion are your GP and the first specialist that you saw. The voluntary organizations (see pages 144–5) may also be able to help.

The second aspect involves your response to the diagnosis. It is not easy for anyone to accept that there is something wrong with them. People who have gone through this experience have said that a person passes through a number of stages after news of this kind. Numbness and disbelief are often followed by anger and sometimes depression before the situation is fully accepted. You may find it helpful to talk this through (see page 30).

Can I be refused another opinion?
No, not really. But your GP may be reluctant to ask another specialist to see you if it is felt that the diagnosis is absolutely certain. Like most professionals, doctors feel that they usually get it right and do not like their authority being challenged. So before asking for another opinion, it's best to analyse what exactly you are unhappy about. Do you really think the diagnosis is wrong or are you resisting the idea that you could have this problem and are anxious about the implications? Talking it over with someone you know well or with another well-informed person such as the health visitor, practice nurse or voluntary organization adviser, may well help. But if you want another opinion, ask for one. And make sure it's the right one.

Points to remember

- A lot of people have a single fit but only some of these have more attacks and are diagnosed as having epilepsy
- To make a diagnosis, doctors need details about the person's medical history and family details as well as accurate eye-witness accounts about what actually happened.
- Tests do not usually make or break the diagnosis of epilepsy
- Even if the fits stop, it can be very difficult to know whether the epilepsy is still present

For more information about:

3 How will having epilepsy affect my life?

After going through the often traumatic experience of having a seizure for the first time, some people are reassured by the expert medical attention they receive and are sometimes glad to be told what they've got. Other people are very frightened at the idea that they are now 'epileptic'.

In this chapter we look at the implications that this diagnosis may have for you, and indicate areas that you need to consider for the future. As in most situations, being forewarned is being forearmed.

. . . .

Should I call myself 'an epileptic'?
It's really up to you. But there are considerable dangers in using this sort of label to describe yourself. You are after all an individual with talents and ambitions. You are not just a walking diagnosis. You also don't know how other people will react to this word. Do they know as much about epilepsy and as much about you, as you do?

On the other hand, you will probably want to find some way of talking about your condition to other people. Saying 'I have epilepsy', 'I have epileptic seizures' or 'I am a person with epilepsy' does not define you in terms of your epilepsy.

Should I tell everyone that I have epilepsy?
Telling people about any medical condition can be very necessary or wildly inappropriate, and this certainly applies to epilepsy. Knowing when to tell what and to whom can be tricky. It all

depends on the circumstances. Close family members are likely to know that something has been happening to you and need reassurance. If there is any real chance of your having fits at school, at work or when out with friends, it seems sensible at least to tell your friends and colleagues what to do. If you do have a fit, then it's less likely to be a problem. Adopting a positive approach to epilepsy is likely to help others to accept it – and you – better.

You may be required to disclose the epilepsy, if, for example, you fill in an application form for a new school, life insurance policy or driving licence. Here you certainly should not lie. When applying for jobs, it's more difficult. Again, don't lie but choose your moment and make sure you know how to put the point across. This is discussed further in Chapter 8 (pages 95–8).

Prognosis and outcome

Will my fits stop or get worse?
The best person to advise you is the doctor who is managing your case. In seven out of ten people seizures will stop usually as a result of simple drug treatment. Only if drug treatment fails initially can the fits get progressively worse, and even in these cases a lot can be done to keep them under reasonable control.

Will my son just grow out of his fits?
This depends on what type of fit he has been having and a number of other things. There are some kinds of fit which always disappear as children get older. These are petit mal absences and benign focal seizures (see pages 47 and 51). They are diagnosed using EEGs. For all other seizure types the outlook may also be very good. Drug treatment is the best way to control attacks in the short term and many children will then stop having them altogether.

Will the drugs get rid of my fits?

Whether drug treatment will work for you depends on a number of factors. The most important is the type of fit that you've had. Also, the cause of your epilepsy can influence the prospects for control. The best person to answer this important question in detail is the doctor who has all the details about your epilepsy.

Having said this, there are some general points which can be made. Early treatment and control of fits seem to result in better control in the long term. The generalized seizures, such as absences, myoclonic and tonic-clonic fits (see pages 47 and 48), generally respond well to drug treatment. Usually about eight out of ten people affected by this type of fit can expect to have no seizures with drug treatment. People who have more than one type of fit tend to experience more difficulty in achieving full control. Partial fits are known to be harder to control than generalized ones, but even in this group, the majority of people can expect drugs to help significantly. For more discussion of the different seizure types, see Chapter 5 (pages 42–53).

Can you tell me what will happen to my epilepsy in the future?

This is a vital question for anyone who has epilepsy. Unfortunately it is a difficult one for doctors to answer. There are no hard-and-fast rules, as every person's condition is different. Gathering information about what happens to people with epilepsy over twenty to thirty years is a difficult task, but studies of this type have tended to give an encouraging picture. In one long-term study, half the people with epilepsy of unknown cause had been free of seizures for five years by the time twenty years had passed after diagnosis. Similarly, about one-third of people with epilepsy as a result of brain damage were also free of seizures.

Can my epilepsy be cured?

When doctors used the word 'cure' they mean that the condition they have treated has completely disappeared and is very unlikely to appear again. This doesn't happen very commonly in epilepsy. None of the drugs which are currently available for epilepsy cure the condition; at best, they control seizures. In a very few people, specialized surgery on the brain (see pages 89–90) can cure epilepsy. Also, in a few people, epilepsy results from disease elsewhere in the body. If this disease can be cured, then the epilepsy is cured along with it.

However, in many people the epilepsy will go into remission, which means that the condition is controlled and seizures have stopped. What is difficult in epilepsy is predicting whether seizures will ever come back. This is why doctors prefer to talk about remission rather than cure.

My son seems to be getting worse each year. Why?
General health and mental abilities are usually not affected by epilepsy. But in some people, a worsening does occur. The possible causes of declining fitness in a person with epilepsy are:

1 The worsening of a disease which is causing the epilepsy
2 Very frequent seizures
3 Another condition which is unrelated to the epilepsy
4 Inappropriate drug treatment

If your son does appear to be getting worse, you should discuss it with your doctor. A full review of your son's condition and treatment is needed. Although sometimes nothing can be done, it is very important to make sure that any cause which can be corrected is attended to.

Will my fits get worse as I get older?
No, not usually. The best way to ensure good control in future is to get fits under complete control as quickly as possible and to keep them fully controlled, even if this means taking medication for a long time. On the other hand, a long period of poor fit-control is likely to make the outlook much less good.

What can I do to prevent further attacks?
Apart from taking treatment there may be little you can do as most fits happen apparently spontaneously. Some people's fits are triggered by specific situations such as alcohol, lack of sleep or flashing lights, and so avoiding these is wise. You can only really find out about these through experience. Further guidance about trigger factors can be found in Chapter 7 (pages 79–84).

Can I die in a fit?
Yes, but this is very rare. Tragically, people can be found dead following an attack. Probably they have choked and not been able to breathe properly as the fit subsides. If there is someone around who knows what to do, the chances of dying in a fit are minimal.

Does this mean I have to have someone with me the whole time?
No, certainly not. Unfortunately the sight of a loved one having a fit is so distressing to some people that it makes them profoundly anxious. Because of their own reaction they feel that the person with epilepsy must always be accompanied. Although this attitude is very understandable, it can lead to intolerable restrictions and overprotection.

Does having epilepsy mean I will die sooner than other people?
Only people with very severe epilepsy or a disease causing the epilepsy have a higher risk of dying earlier than do those people without epilepsy.

First aid

What should I do when my son has a grand mal fit?
The main thing you need to do when your son has a grand mal or tonic-clonic seizure (see page 47) is to make sure he doesn't injure himself. There is nothing you can do to stop the seizure or make it stop sooner. So you should just let the seizure run its course.

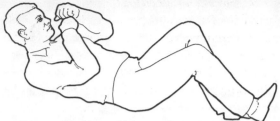

Remove any objects which may cause injury.

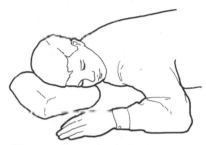

Place a cushion under the head.

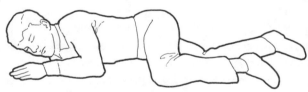

Try to get the person on to his side.
Help the person to move to a comfortable position when ready.

The main aim should be to prevent injury and place the person in a comfortable position, either lying or sitting. Ideally the person should be placed in the recovery position.

What to do when someone has a fit in which they fall

If your son falls to the ground, gently turn him on to his side as soon as you can. You may want to put a pillow or something soft under his head to protect it. Don't try to interfere with the movements of his body, but do make sure there is nothing around against which he is likely to hit his arms or legs. Don't try to force anything between his teeth. You could loosen any tight clothing.

Some people go rather blue around the lips during a seizure. This is called *cyanosis*. It happens because breathing has been interrupted during the fit. Once it is over, normal colour will return quickly. But if it doesn't, check inside the mouth to make sure that nothing is blocking the airway.

When your son's seizure stops, just sit with him until he wakes up. People often feel very drowsy, confused or irritable when waking from a seizure. They need to know someone is there but don't need a lot of conversation or questions.

What should I do to help people having other kinds of seizure?
The principles of first aid for all seizures are the same – try to prevent the person from coming to harm without interfering too much. For example, if someone has the kind of seizure where he walks around in a dazed way, then you should just follow him and lead him gently away from any dangerous situation. If an injury occurs, this may need separate first aid or other treatment.

When my daughter has a fit, how long do I wait before I call the doctor or the ambulance?
You should discuss with your doctor at an early stage what you should do if your daughter has more attacks. The advice will vary according to the type of fit, the circumstances in which they occur and your ability to cope. Parents can give extra treatment which will help to stop the fit if it is unusually prolonged (see page 43 for more details). But most fits are quite short and do no great harm.

The same applies to adults with epilepsy. It's a good idea to discuss the situation with the doctor, so that everyone is clear about what to do. Your local epilepsy group (see pages 144–5) may also be helpful in this area.

Do I need to go to hospital every time I have a fit?
No, you don't. It's not necessary. But it may be very difficult to convince people who do not know you well that this is the case. Well-meaning people often call an ambulance if they see someone having a fit, usually because they do not feel confident to deal with the situation themselves. Once the ambulance has been called, the ambulance staff usually feel they have to take you to hospital, so you can be checked over by a doctor.

Only if you have been badly injured in a fit, if one fit follows another, or if recovery is more delayed than usual, should a visit to hospital be strictly necessary. But it's equally important that those people who are likely to be with you if you have an attack, know what to do and feel confident to deal with the situation. They may need educating and you can play an important part in this.

Daily life

In this short section we look at some of the areas of your life that may be immediately affected by the start of epilepsy. How it will actually affect you as a person with epilepsy or as a family member will depend on many things, including particularly how quickly the fits stop. More details about all these issues are given in Chapters 7, 8 and 9.

Since starting epilepsy, my son has been very low in himself. What can I do to help?
Having fits for the first time and being diagnosed as having epilepsy is a very traumatic experience. It's quite easy to think that having epilepsy has ruined your life. Some people with epilepsy say that it's like a bereavement. What is lost is not a friend or a member of the

family but part of yourself, often your self-esteem.

So a period of being low, even depressed, is quite understandable, and it often helps to talk over the feelings and try to look objectively at the situation. This is easier said than done and expert counselling may be invaluable at this time, not only for the individual but for the whole family. Your GP, the hospital doctor or the voluntary organizations may be able to help you find a counsellor.

Will there be problems at school now that my daughter has epilepsy?
How to approach the situation depends on whether your daughter is at primary or secondary school. At primary school, your daughter's teacher certainly needs to know about her history of seizures. Hiding her epilepsy could result in her being exposed to danger (such as being allowed to swim unsupervised). In secondary school, the best person to talk to initially is the head teacher, and you should then devise a plan for telling others as necessary. If your daughter continues to have fits, even for a short period, the school may want to take extra safety precautions in activities like games and science subjects.

Sadly, some teachers know little about epilepsy and may want to restrict your daughter's activities too much. This should be resisted, but you may need professional help from your GP, specialist, school nurse or community paediatrician. The voluntary organizations can also help by providing direct advice to the school. They have excellent leaflets, posters and videos made especially for teachers. School problems are looked at again on pages 124–7.

Can I continue to drive?
No, you must not. Once the diagnosis of epilepsy is made, you must inform the Driving and Vehicle Licensing Centre (DVLC) in Swansea what has happened to you. Telephone them on 0792 30 4482 and quote your driving licence number. Your licence will be withdrawn and the DVLC will inform you of this. If you want to appeal against this decision, you have to apply to a magistrates' court within

thirty days. You will probably need the help of a solicitor to do this, who may in turn need to ask the opinion of a specialist. In practice you can first appeal to the DVLC who may ask for the opinion of its Honorary Medical Advisory Panel.

If you continue to drive having been advised not to by a doctor, then you do so illegally and will not be covered by your insurance.

You can reapply for your licence once you have been completely free of fits for two years from the date of the last attack. If you only have fits while asleep you can reapply for a licence three years after the first sleep attack, even if your attacks have continued. All types of disturbance due to epilepsy, including jerks and auras (see pages 47 and 51), count as attacks for the purposes of these regulations. Driving is discussed again on pages 98–102.

Can I continue to play sport, swim and ride a bike?
You mustn't think of yourself as being ill and give up these activities for that reason. However, you must also consider the risks that would be involved if you had an attack while swimming alone, climbing a rock face or cycling in traffic. It could well be the end of you and possibly be dangerous to others. It's a question of weighing up the risks. This is not easy and requires some thought. You must be careful to avoid unnecessary risks. Having a friend who agrees to keep an eye on you is helpful. The Americans call this the 'buddy' system. Leaders of activities should be informed about your epilepsy and what to do if you have a fit. If you do decide to give up an activity even temporarily, it's as well to find another to take its place.

Can I continue to have sex?
Yes, you can. Some people are understandably worried about the possibility of having an attack when they are making love. Sexual activity doesn't bring on attacks so the chances of this happening to you must be very small. Even if it did happen, no one would come to any great harm.

Will having epilepsy affect my job prospects?
It could. Some occupations, such as driving heavy goods vehicles (lorries, etc.) and public service vehicles (buses, etc.), are barred by law to people who have had seizures. Working in some professions, for example nursing and teaching, can be a problem unless the attacks have been completely controlled for some years. Factory jobs, particularly those involving working with heavy machinery, working alone for long periods, at heights or near open water, are often considered too dangerous. School-leavers who continue to have seizures will often benefit from seeing the specialist careers advisor at school. All government training schemes for young people are open to those with epilepsy (see pages 95–8).

Should I tell my employer?
Fortunately most employers will respond sympathetically and there may be good reasons why yours should be informed. But before telling your employer you should consider whether the fact that you have had fits is relevant to your job. It could be in three ways. First, if you have to have time off work for hospital appointments, your employer might want to know why. Second, continuing with your present job might be too dangerous both to yourself and others. Third, you could have a fit at work. If none of these applies to you, then you may consider it sensible to wait and see what happens. You might, after all, never have another attack. If you are asked directly about your state of health you must not lie, otherwise you are breaking the Health and Safety at Work Act. This means that your employer could dismiss you, and you could not claim unfair dismissal at an industrial tribunal.

What do I do if my employer wants to sack me?
Get expert advice. Your GP and hospital consultant will be able to advise you, and you should involve your trade union or professional association, if you have one. You can also get help from the Employment Medical Advisory Service and the voluntary organizations (see pages 144–50). Employment problems are looked at again on pages 95–8.

Points to remember

- Calling yourself 'an epileptic' is using a label, but you need to find some way of talking about your epilepsy.
- Telling other people that you have epilepsy may be important for your own safety.
- School-teachers must be informed about a child who has a history of fits.
- You need a plan for dealing with fits, agreed with your doctor.
- You must not drive and you must inform the DVLC about the fact that you have epilepsy.
- Drug treatment is the best way to ensure complete fit control.
- Most activities can be continued, given proper precautions, but some may have to be discontinued temporarily.
- Job prospects can be affected because of epilepsy.

For more information about:

– Treatment, see pages 34–41, 54–76 and 85–91.
– Seizure types, see pages 45–53.
– Employment, see pages 95–8 and 134–5.
– Relationships, see pages 115–23
– Schooling, see pages 124–7.
– Leisure, see pages 135–6.

4 Why do I have to take this medicine?

Most people with epilepsy take medication for a long time. The shortest period is usually two years and some people need to take it for the rest of their lives. Knowing a lot about the drug treatment for epilepsy is therefore important and not something that only doctors should know about.

In this chapter we explore some of the common problems that you may encounter with your treatment. The first section deals with starting treatment, and the second with how you can manage your treatment most effectively. Chapter 6 looks at the different drugs in more detail, and stopping treatment is considered in Chapter 8.

. . . .

Starting treatment

How will drug treatment help?
When starting you on an anti-epileptic drug, your doctor has two broad aims in mind: to control your seizures and at the same time to cause no side-effects, or as few as possible.

How do the drugs work?
The exact way in which anti-epileptic drugs work is not known, except in the case of one new drug, vigabatrin (Sabril). Basically, the drugs are thought to interfere with the passage of electrical messages between brain cells – either by altering brain chemicals, or making cells less likely to 'fire'. Vigabatrin is known to increase

the level of a brain chemical called GABA which acts to stop brain cells firing.

Why did my doctor choose the drug which I'm taking now?
Some types of seizure respond better to one type of drug than another, so this will guide your doctor's choice. If there are several drugs which are effective in a particular type of seizure, the choice of drug may then be on the basis of side-effects, the number of doses which must be taken a day, how easily the dose is adjusted, and so on.

Response to drugs can vary a lot, so sometimes 'trial and error' is needed to find a drug which both works well and agrees with you.

Why am I taking this particular dose of drug?
The right dose of drug is the one which controls your seizures without giving you unpleasant side-effects. As with the right drug, the right dose may take a little while to establish. The first dosage level is usually a low one. Your doctor will then want to know if you have had any seizures or side-effects after a period on this dose. If you have more attacks, then the dose will probably be increased.

A blood test may be used to measure the level of the drug in your blood. This can serve as a guide as to whether you are getting too little or too much of the drug. But for some drugs, blood tests are not useful (see page 58).

What is monotherapy?
This term is used to describe treatment with just one drug. Occasionally, a person will need more than one drug. This is called polytherapy.

How often will I need to see my doctor now that treatment has started?
In the beginning, you will probably need to go to see the specialist every few weeks in order to report any side-effects or fits. Once the best drug and dose for you are found, regular checks are needed

every few months. Once treatment is running smoothly, checks can be made once or twice yearly. Your GP may also ask to see you if you need repeat prescriptions from the surgery.

How often do I need to have blood tests?
Tests for levels of the drug in your blood are not necessary at every visit. They are used to guide the correct dose when you are starting certain drugs. For example, tests are particularly useful with phenytoin but much less useful with sodium valproate. Such tests are then usually only needed if you have any side-effects or if seizures are still occurring.

Taking your medicine

I really don't want to take treatment at all. Do I have to?
No, you don't. It's your decision. But medicines are the best way, in most people, to control attacks completely. If you decide not to take treatment you may not find your specialist or GP is very sympathetic if you have attacks.

Do I have to take my tablets with food?
No. Epilepsy drugs can be taken at any time.

If I am late with a dose, does this matter?
Not usually, no. Some people with fits that are very difficult to control find that the exact timing of their tablets is important. But for most people, spacing the tablets out at approximately regular intervals as prescribed by your doctor is good enough.

If I forget a dose, what should I do?
Missing a single dose isn't likely to do you much harm. However, it's important to keep the intake of your drugs as regular as possible. So if you miss one dose, take it as soon as you remember, or add it to the dose you take next time.

What do I do if I get ill?
You should keep taking your medicine as usual. If you are vomiting, you may have to wait until this has stopped before starting your epilepsy treatment again. If this is only a matter of a few hours, you shouldn't come to too much harm. If you cannot take your epilepsy drug for more than twelve hours, you need advice from your GP. If you get severe diarrhoea, drink plenty of fluids and take your epilepsy medicine as usual. It should not be necessary to alter the dose of your drug.

Some young children are prone to fits if they get a high temperature, and other remedies are sometimes advised, such as tepid sponging and paracetamol.

If you need emergency treatment for another illness, you must always tell the doctor that you are on epilepsy treatment. A card with the name of the drug and dosage can be useful. An example is shown in the diagram on page 38.

I really have difficulty remembering to take my tablets. What can I do about this?
It isn't easy for anyone to remember to take medicine regularly over a long period. Most people forget from time to time. If you are having a lot of difficulty it may be that your tablet schedule could be simplified by your doctor so that, say, you only have to take it once or twice a day. Leaving your pill bottle by your toothbrush is a good way of reminding yourself (although you must be careful of safety if there are children around).

Devices such as pill dispensers can also be very helpful. These can be bought from a pharmacist.

My daughter always relies on me to give her the tablets. Is this a good idea?
Young children obviously need supervision over medicines. But the sooner your daughter takes responsibility for her own drugs the better it is for her, even if this means anxiety for you, and perhaps the occasional missed dose.

NSE
NATIONAL
SOCIETY
FOR EPILEPSY

THE OWNER OF THIS CARD HAS EPILEPSY

NAME: A. PATIENT
ADDRESS: ✎✎✎✎
Tel. no. 000 0000

In case of emergency please contact:
Name: MRS A. PATIENT
Address: ✎✎✎✎
Tel. no. 000 0000

GUIDANCE ON THE MANAGEMENT OF EPILEPTIC FITS INSIDE

My fits usually take the following form:

1. I LOOK BLANK AND RATHER PALE. I'M NOT ABLE TO RESPOND AND MAY WANDER ABOUT. (COMPLEX PARTIAL FIT)
2. VERY OCCASIONALLY THIS LEADS TO A MAJOR ATTACK IN WHICH I STIFFEN AND FALL AND HAVE A CONVULSION.
3.

Other information: AFTER A MAJOR FIT I USUALLY RECOVER QUICKLY BUT MAY NOT BE ENTIRELY SURE WHERE I AM FOR 20 MINUTES OR SO.

I USUALLY TAKE 20 MINUTES TO RECOVER FULLY.

MR. A. PATIENT is under my care for the treatment of epilepsy, and requires to take the following medication regularly:

NAME OF DRUG	TOTAL DAILY DOSE
CARBAMAZEPINE	1000 MG

Name, address, tel. no. of hospital doctor 000 0000
DR BROWN

G.P's name, address, tel. no. 000 0000
DR SMITH

Dr's. Signature: P.Bur Date: 4.4.91

Epilepsy drug card

What do I do if I run out of tablets?

This is potentially very dangerous and you should always make sure that you have enough. Never stop taking your medicines abruptly as this may cause *status epilepticus* (see page 52). If you do run out and are away from home, you can consult any GP to get some more, or as a last resort go to a local hospital casualty department. But you won't be very popular! Some people with epilepsy recommend that you keep a small spare supply of tablets at home just in case you run out.

Do I have to pay for my epilepsy drugs?

No, you don't. All drugs for epilepsy can be dispensed without a prescription charge unless you are being treated privately, when you will have to pay the full costs of the drugs. In order to get your medicines free, however, you have to get an exemption certificate. You need to fill in Form P11 which you can get from your GP, your chemist or the Social Security office. It has to be countersigned by your doctor.

Is it safe for me to take other medicines that I can buy from the chemist?

Yes, it is safe, although it's quite a good idea to let the chemist know you take epilepsy drugs, just to make sure. And always read what it says on the package before you take the medicine. But no commonly available remedies should cause any problems.

Will taking epilepsy drugs affect my sex life?

Very occasionally this can happen. We know very little about the effect of epilepsy drugs on women's hormones and how this could affect their sex drive. In men, we know a bit more but this is largely the result of laboratory tests of hormone levels rather than studies on how these might affect how you feel. If you think that the drugs are a problem to you in this way you really need expert advice. It's not something that many doctors think to ask about, so you may have to mention it yourself.

Can my doctor prescribe other drugs if I need them?
Yes. Most other drugs are no problem. There are a few medicines that do not combine well with epilepsy drugs and extra precautions are necessary. The only commonly prescribed drug which you have to be careful about is the contraceptive pill. This can be made less effective by some epilepsy drugs (phenytoin, carbamazepine and phenobarbitone/primidone). For more details, see sections on the individual drugs, pages 61–70. For more information on the Pill, see pages 63, 65 and 66. You should always tell any doctor or dentist you consult that you take epilepsy drugs, and it's a good idea to have the names and doses written down.

Will I be able to get my usual medicines if I go abroad?
You will probably be able to obtain the same drugs (unless you are going to a developing country) but not necessarily in the form that you are used to. The name, colour and shape of the tablets may be different and also the dose may vary. It's safer to take all the medicine that you will need with you unless you are going to be abroad for a long time.

Some customs officials can be difficult if they find you are carrying a lot of pills and so it's a good idea to have a note from your doctor or pharmacist confirming that you need to have them. Experienced travellers who have epilepsy recommend you keep a supply of tablets in your hand luggage in case you are delayed or your baggage goes astray.

If you are planning on living abroad, you should register with a doctor there and take some medical information about your condition with you. Your specialist in the UK should be able to tell you if your drugs are available where you are going. The *Traveller's Handbook*, published by the International Bureau for Epilepsy (see page 138), also has a lot of useful information.

Points to remember

- The decision to take or not to take treatment is yours.
- Regular spacing of the medicine as prescribed throughout the day gives the best chance of fit control.
- A missed dose should be made up as soon as possible.
- Children with epilepsy should look after their own medicine as early as possible.
- Never run out of medicine. It's extremely dangerous.
- Other medicines can normally be taken quite safely with epilepsy drugs.
- Special precautions are needed with the contraceptive pill.

For more information about:

- Status epilepticus, see pages 52 and 126.
- Epilepsy drugs and other medicines, see pages 61–70.
- Stopping treatment, see pages 92–4.
- Travel, see page 136.

5   Epilepsy in perspective

In this chapter we look at information about the patterns of fits in the general population and the different groups of people who develop epilepsy. We then turn to look at the different types of seizure – what they are called and what the names mean.

. . . .

Epilepsy in the general population

Am I the only one with epilepsy?
Actually, epilepsy is one of the most common disorders involving the brain. In the UK, and in most other countries, about one in every 200 people has epilepsy. Studies have indicated that about fifty out of every 100,000 people in the general population have epilepsy diagnosed each year.

The number of people getting epilepsy each year is called the *incidence* of epilepsy. The number of people who have the condition at any one time is referred to as the *prevalence* of epilepsy.

Are more people getting epilepsy?
There are no signs that the number of people developing epilepsy each year – the *incidence* – is increasing. It's often difficult to know precisely how many people are affected, because some people choose to hide the fact. However, as attitudes to epilepsy have changed, it seems that more people have become willing to discuss their condition. In developed countries, improvements in health

care this century have probably reduced the amount of epilepsy resulting from brain damage occurring at birth or soon after birth. But as we still don't know the cause in the vast majority of people, there has as yet been no real progress in reducing the incidence of epilepsy overall.

What about children? Do they often have epilepsy?
Epilepsy often begins during childhood. About half the individuals who are going to develop epilepsy start to have fits before they are adults. In the other half, the condition appears during the late teenage or adult years.

Some fits occur only in children. Fits during a feverish illness, called *febrile convulsions*, are quite common in infants and pre-school children. About three out of every 100 children have a febrile convulsion. About half of these never experience another fit, and the tendency to febrile convulsions disappears quite quickly, usually by the age of five. Such children are not considered to have epilepsy.

You say that febrile convulsions are not epilepsy, but my son's doctor wants to put him on medicine because he is having these. Will this help him?
Yes, it probably will. But there are a number of things which you need to consider first. After the first febrile convulsion, one in two children will not have any more. Even for children who have had a second convulsion, regular medicine is not usually advised, but parents will be asked to give treatment to their child as soon as a fever starts. This aims to cool them down by sponging with tepid water and giving paracetamol.

If the fits are very long, if they are repeated, or if the doctor is worried that they might do the child harm, then specific treatment can be given by parents to stop the fit. This is in the form of diazepam (Valium) given as a tablet, syrup or as a suppository. The parents may be asked to inject the diazepam into the child's rectum using a special tube (see page 44). Your doctor will advise you about the best way of treating your son and the dose of diazepam to be given.

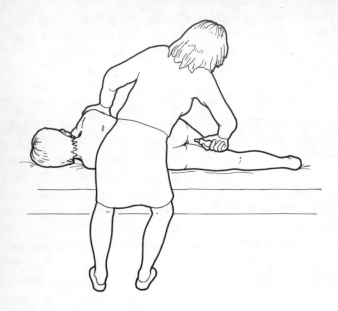

Injecting diazepam via the rectum

Only if this method is not effective in controlling the fits, will doctors usually recommend daily treatment with medicine. At the moment the choice of drug lies between phenobarbitone and sodium valproate (Epilim). Both are effective in controlling febrile seizures but both have unpleasant side-effects in some children (see pages 66 and 67), and treatment needs to be continued for at least two years. So the whole business needs discussion and careful thought.

Is epilepsy more common in men than in women?
Epilepsy does occur slightly more often in men than in women. The reasons for this are not really known, but some researchers have suggested that this is due to the fact that men are more liable to head injury than women.

Are boys more likely to have epilepsy than girls?
The boy–girl ratios vary according to the type of fit. For example, febrile convulsions are more common in boys, while absences (see pages 47–9) are more often seen in girls.

If a baby is born prematurely, is it likely to develop epilepsy?
The brain of a newborn baby is very sensitive. This sensitivity is even more marked if the baby is born prematurely. Periods without enough oxygen, severe infections, or periods of low blood sugar can all affect the baby's brain, and all these things can happen to a premature baby. Doctors sometimes refer to this kind of event as an 'insult' to the brain. Any insult to the brain can increase the chance of epilepsy developing, but it won't always happen by any means.

My daughter, who's now five, had some fits just after she was born. Does this mean she'll have epilepsy later?
Your daughter had what we call *neonatal seizures*. These are often due to some chemical imbalance within the baby's body and once this has been corrected, the fits stop. Provided that she has no other signs of problems with her brain, then you shouldn't expect her to get epilepsy later in life.

Different types of seizure

Does everyone with epilepsy have the same sorts of fit?
No. There are a number of types of seizure and someone with epilepsy may experience only one type of attack, or several.

In recent years an internationally agreed classification of epileptic seizures has been devised. The discussion which follows is based on the most recent system, and this is illustrated in the diagram on page 46. Many people still use the old names, like grand mal and petit mal. Although most people will understand what you mean by them, the new names are much more accurate and informative.

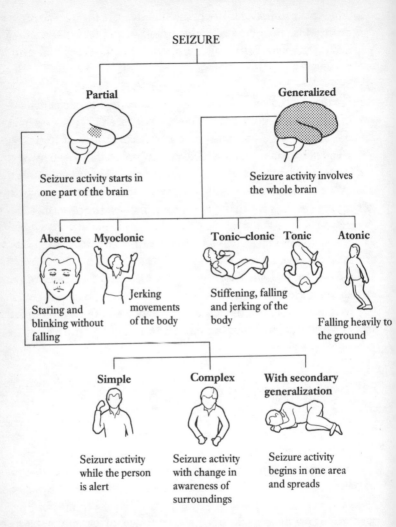

Classification of seizures

How does my doctor know what kind of fit I have?
The most important information used to classify seizures is a description of what actually happened to you during the fit. Information from your EEG and perhaps from other tests may also help to label your seizures correctly.

I have generalized seizures. What does that mean?
This term is used to refer to seizures which begin in both sides of the brain at the same time. They start very abruptly and the person affected has no warning. There are five types of generalized seizure. The best known of these is the *tonic-clonic seizure* (sometimes also called grand mal). The person suddenly blacks out and falls to the ground. The body stiffens (the tonic phase) followed by jerking movements of the arms and legs (the clonic phase). The tonic and clonic phases usually last for about one to two minutes. The person may be unconscious for several minutes after the seizure has finished, and upon waking is often drowsy and confused. Some people then fall asleep for several hours.

If only the stiffening of the body occurs, without the rapid jerking movements, the seizures are called *tonic*.

What are the other types of generalized seizure?
Absence seizures, also known as petit mal, occur in childhood. Usually, the child stares and loses awareness of his or her surroundings for several seconds, but does not fall to the ground. There may be blinking and some movements of the face. The child then suddenly wakes and has no memory of the last few seconds.

If the brief interruption of awareness is accompanied by jerking movements of the face, arms or legs, the term *complex absence* is used.

In *atonic seizures*, sometimes called drop attacks, the person suddenly loses the normal tone in the body, falling heavily to the ground, but is able to get up again almost immediately.

Sudden jerking movements of the body are termed *myoclonic*

seizures. The arm, head and trunk may jerk, sometimes so forcefully that the person falls to the ground.

One doctor said my son has petit mal, and another said he has absences. Who is right?

They are both right, as these two names refer to the same type of fit. The names of seizures can be a bit confusing because, over the years, the terminology has changed. The new and old terms used to describe seizures are set out in the following table. (It's better for everyone to use the new terms as they are more accurate.)

New and old names for seizures

NEW	OLD
absence	petit mal
myoclonic	minor motor
clonic	grand mal
tonic	grand mal
tonic-clonic	grand mal
atonic seizures	akinetic, drop attacks, minor motor
simple partial seizures	focal or local seizures
with motor symptoms	focal motor or Jacksonian
with sensory symptoms	focal sensory
complex partial	psychomotor seizures
	temporal lobe seizures

If you don't understand the names your doctor uses, make sure you ask. It is important that you are both talking about the same thing when you discuss your son's attacks. Sometimes people find their own way of labelling their seizures (such as 'big attacks' and 'little attacks') and agree to use those terms with their doctor. This is fine as long as you always see the same doctor, but learning the proper name for your son's kind of fit can avoid confusion.

Can adults have absences?

Absences always start in childhood but sometimes they persist as the person grows older. So for this reason adults can have absences. But attacks which start in an adult and may look like absences are almost certainly complex partial seizure of a very minor type.

My doctor said I have partial seizures. What did she mean?

This name refers to seizures which occur when the epileptic discharge is limited to one part of the brain. Partial seizures can then be further divided into two groups, complex and simple.

Complex partial seizures occur when the person's awareness of his or her surroundings is affected during a seizure. In simple partial seizures the patient is fully aware of what is happening. Warnings are quite common before partial seizures and the onset can be gradual. Full recovery after the attack may take some minutes, although needing to sleep afterwards is unusual. Some people with partial seizures say they feel very drained afterwards. In some people a partial seizure can develop into a full-blown tonic-clonic seizure, a process technically known as *secondary generalization*.

Are all partial seizures the same?

No. The symptoms of a partial seizure depend on where the unusual brain activity is occurring. For example, if the discharge begins in the part of the brain controlling movement, the person will experience unusual movements during an attack. A lot of other experiences can occur in partial seizures, such as pins and needles sensations, dizziness or funny tastes and smells – it all depends on where in the brain the seizure is happening. You can see this better by looking at the diagram.

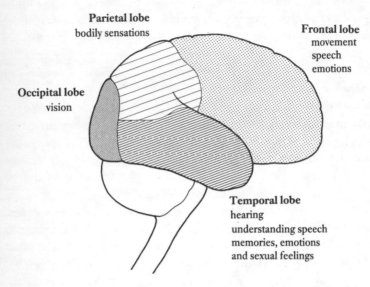

Parietal lobe
bodily sensations

Frontal lobe
movement
speech
emotions

Occipital lobe
vision

Temporal lobe
hearing
understanding speech
memories, emotions
and sexual feelings

What happens during a seizure depends on the part of the brain affected.

Different areas of the brain

Sometimes these symptoms may be quite complicated. For example, if the seizure involves a part of the brain called the temporal lobe, the person may experience what is called déjà vu. This is a sense that what is happening to you has all happened before. Emotions such as fear or pleasure can also occur.

In the course of a seizure, or after the seizure has finished, the person affected may perform actions without knowing what he or she is doing. These actions are called *automatisms*. Examples of automatisms include smacking the lips, repeated swallowing, or fumbling movement of the hands. Sometimes more complex automatisms take place. For example, a person may undress, walk out of the house, begin to cook or search for objects – all in an inappropriate way. Generally, automatisms last less than five minutes.

Various combinations of the symptoms may occur during a seizure, but in any one person the pattern of events is usually quite similar each time a seizure occurs.

My son has been diagnosed as having benign focal seizures. What does this mean?

Focal attacks that have a very good outlook in children have been recognized only recently. They often occur while the child is asleep. In the most common type of attack, the child gets repeated twitching of one side of the face and the arm on the same side. Occasionally the leg is affected as well. If the fit occurs while awake the child may be unable to speak during the attack but does not go unconscious. If the fits only occur during sleep and are infrequent, the doctor may recommend that no treatment is given. You can expect the attacks to stop completely before your son has reached the age of twenty.

Do people get a warning before a fit?

Some people do. This is because their seizures begin in one part of the brain before spreading to involve a larger area of the brain. This spread may be quite slow, giving plenty of warning that a fit is about to occur, or it may be very rapid. These warning symptoms are called an *aura* and are part of the fit itself.

Warnings vary tremendously, however. For example, some people may experience tightness in the throat and a feeling of dizziness just before falling to the ground with a tonic-clonic seizure. Other people who have auras report a rising sensation starting in the pit of the stomach; others hear noises. Auras can happen just before tonic-clonic or complex partial seizures and they show that the fit starts in one part of the brain.

People will sometimes notice a change in themselves for several days before a fit. This varies, but may consist of irritability, a feeling of depression, or just a sense of something 'building up'. This is not called an aura but is often referred to as the *prodrome* of a seizure.

Why does my wife's speech change when she has a fit?
Speech can be affected during seizures if the disturbance involves the areas of the brain which control speech. Sometimes people cannot speak at all for a brief period, or their words are slurred or difficult to understand. People who experience this say that it is a very frustrating and upsetting experience. Occasionally people may say odd or irrelevant things when they are confused after a seizure.

What is status epilepticus?
This term describes the occurrence of a number of seizures without recovery in between. If the person is having tonic-clonic seizures, status epilepticus is a medical emergency which requires very active treatment by doctors to stop the seizures. Fortunately only about three out of 100 people with this type of seizure ever experience status epilepticus. It may be brought on by such things as sudden withdrawal of epileptic drugs, other illness or excessive alcohol. Often, however, there is no clear cause.

Other types of status, for example *absence status*, can also occur, but usually only in people with other handicaps (see page 126). This is not quite such a medical emergency but requires expert management as it can be difficult to diagnose.

Points to remember

- Epilepsy is quite a common condition in the general population.
- There are many types of seizure, and they may have more than one name.
- Generalized seizures begin in both sides of the brain at the same time.
- Partial seizures begin in one part of the brain.
- What happens during a seizure depends on which areas of the brain are affected.

For more information about:

Different types of seizure

Epilepsy: a practical guide to coping by L. Sander and P. Thompson (Crowood Health Guides), chapter 1 (paperback for lay people).

Epilepsy, ed. A. Hopkins (Chapman and Hall Medical), chapter 3, 'The different types of epileptic seizure and the international classification of epileptic seizures and of epileptic syndromes' by Fritz Dreifuss (textbook for doctors).

6 Drugs for treating epilepsy

Drug treatment plays a very important role in epilepsy. To manage your treatment well, you need to understand as much as you can about the drugs, why they are used and what to do if there are problems. Unfortunately no drug is perfect. They all have their advantages and disadvantages which have to be weighed up for each different person.

This chapter covers some general questions about drug treatment, and then looks a little more closely at the most frequently used drugs. If you have questions which are not answered in this chapter, your doctor should be able to answer them for you.

. . . .

What are the drugs used to treat epilepsy?
There are a number of anti-epileptic drugs (see following table). The four 'first line' drugs are the drugs most commonly used. The 'second line' drugs are less commonly prescribed in the UK, usually because they are used in special situations. Drugs can be prescribed by either the chemical or brand name.

Why do drugs have more than one name?
Drugs have a chemical (or generic) name as well as a brand name. Thus carbamazepine is the generic name, and Tegretol its trade name in the UK. Sometimes trade names vary from country to country, but the generic name always stays the same. It is a good idea for you to know both names of the drug or drugs that you take.

Anti-epileptic drugs

CHEMICAL NAME	BRAND NAME(S)
First line drugs	
Phenytoin	Epanutin
Ethosuximide	Emeside, Zarontin
Sodium valproate	Epilim
Carbamazepine	Tegretol
Second line drugs	
Phenobarbitone	Luminal
Primidone	Mysoline
Diazepam	Valium
Clonazepam	Rivotril
Clobazam	Frisium
Vigabatrin	Sabril

Who makes the drugs?
Generally, a drug is produced and tested by one pharmaceutical company. At this stage, the company owns the patent and gives it a brand name (such as Valium). Once the patent runs out, it may be made and sold under its generic name, or under a different brand name by other companies.

Why are there all these different drugs?
There are a number of reasons why different drugs are used to treat epilepsy. First, the drugs can vary in their effects on different types of seizure. In generalized tonic-clonic seizures, phenytoin (Epanutin), carbamazepine (Tegretol), sodium valproate (Epilim) and phenobarbitone are all effective. In partial seizures, phenytoin, carbamazepine, sodium valproate, phenobarbitone and primidone (Mysoline) have all been used successfully, although many doctors would use carbamazepine first in complex partial seizures. A new drug, vigabatrin (Sabril) has also been shown to be good at

controlling partial seizures. In absence seizures, ethosuximide (Zarontin) or sodium valproate are clearly the most effective drugs. Clonazepam (Rivotril) is often used in myoclonus. The doses and uses of the 'first line' drugs are shown in the following table.

Dose range and use of first line anti-epileptic drugs

DRUG	DOSE RANGE		SEIZURE TYPES
Phenytoin	Adults	150–600 mg/day*	Partial
	Children	5–15 mg/kg/day**	Generalized tonic-clonic
Carbamazepine	Adults	400–1800 mg/day	Partial
	Children	10–30 mg/kg/day	Generalized tonic-clonic
Sodium Valproate	Adults	600–3000 mg/day	Partial
	Children	20–30 mg/kg/day	Generalized tonic-clonic
			Absence
			Myoclonus
Ethosuximide	Adults	500–1500 mg/day	Absence
	Children	10–15 mg/kg/day	

*mg/day refers to the amount of drug (measured in milligrams) taken in twenty-four hours.
**in children, dose is usually calculated on the basis of the child's weight. Thus a child will be prescribed a certain number of milligrams per kilogram of body weight in a twenty-four hour period.

Side-effects

What side-effects can I expect to get?
Hopefully, you won't get any side-effects. But different drugs have different side-effects, and one drug may suit one person but disagree with another. So it is helpful to have a range of drugs to

choose from. The various types of side-effect are shown in the table below.

In the short term, all the epilepsy drugs can make you drowsy or unsteady on your feet if the dose is too high for you. Some people even feel sleepy on a drug if the dose is really low. All the drugs can also produce a rash but this is most common with carbamazepine.

Some side-effects are not seen immediately, however, and these long-term effects can be quite a problem as the connection between the symptom and the drug may be missed.

It's always rather frightening to read a long list of side-effects which the drug you are taking can produce. These lists are drawn up over many years reporting the experiences of a lot of people. By law, drug manufacturers have to list all the side-effects that have been reported with their drug. The side-effects mentioned here are those which have occurred fairly often. But even so, the drugs are still pretty safe and most people can take them without getting any severe problems. Nearly all the side-effects can be minimized if the number of drugs taken is kept to one, or two at the most.

Some side-effects of anti-epileptic drugs

	SIDE-EFFECT	DRUG RESPONSIBLE
Short term	Unsteadiness Drowsiness Confusion	All when dose is too high
	Rash	All, but most often carbamazepine
Long term	Problems with memory, alertness and concentration	phenobarbitone phenytoin
	Irritability and overactivity in children	phenobarbitone vigabatrin
	Enlargement of gums ⎫ Acne ⎭	phenytoin

It's important to realize that these side-effects are only seen in some people who take anti-epileptic drugs. More details are given about the side-effects of each of the drugs as we look at them individually.

Will a blood test tell whether I am getting side-effects?
A blood test may help the doctor know whether your symptoms are likely to be due to your drug dosage. But it depends which drug you are taking. Blood tests measuring the amount of the drug in your blood are not helpful with all the epilepsy drugs. The usefulness of blood tests with the different drugs is shown below.

Value of blood tests for the different drugs

DRUG	NEED FOR BLOOD TESTS
Phenytoin	Essential
Carbamazepine	Useful
Ethosuximide	Useful
Phenobarbitone	Sometimes useful
Primidone Sodium valproate Clonazepam Vigabatrin	Not often useful

My drug is giving me side-effects. What should I do?
It depends what sort of side-effects you are getting. All drugs prescribed for epilepsy have side-effects and these can be mild or serious and sometimes they wear off and sometimes they don't.

If the side-effects are bearable, it's best to keep taking the medicine at the same dose and tell your doctor at your next appointment. If they are severe, you need to get urgent advice from the doctor who prescribed the drug. Your treatment may need changing but don't just stop taking the drug without consulting your doctor.

Balancing seizure control with side-effects can become quite difficult. There is often a 'trade-off' between experiencing seizures and having no side-effects, or having side effects and no seizures. You may need to make the final decision which you prefer – although it is always advisable to ask your doctor's opinion and go into the options thoroughly.

The drug makes me feel sleepy. Will this wear off?
It may do. All epilepsy drugs can cause drowsiness because the drugs are acting on the brain. The newer compounds are less likely to do this and it may be that a small reduction in dose will help. But it's usually worth waiting a few weeks to see what happens.

Do the drugs have any long-term effects?
Yes, some of the drugs, particularly the older ones like pheno-barbitone, and phenytoin, can have long term side-effects (see pages 63 and 67). Most people taking one of the newer drugs, such as sodium valproate or carbamazepine, shouldn't experience any bad effects over a long period of time. It is too early to say much about the long-term effects of vigabatrin.

My daughter has become very irritable since starting treatment. Is it the drug that's doing it?
It may be. Phenobarbitone is particularly connected with changes in behaviour in young children and so it's not used so much now. Any of the drugs can cause moodiness but there may be other reasons as well. Your daughter may be feeling very fed up with the whole business and resent having epilepsy and having to take treatment. But this is an important observation which you should share with your daughter's doctor.

Will the medicine affect my daughter's progress at school?
Learning can be affected by epilepsy drugs but the more modern ones such as carbamazepine and sodium valproate are less harmful in

this respect. Vigabatrin is too new to know much about its effects on children at school. Keeping the dose to the minimum that controls the fits is important with all drugs to avoid harmful effects.

I feel that I am poisoning my son by giving him this medicine. Am I harming him?

Many parents have quite reasonable fears about their children taking medicines over a long period of time. Some feel that they would much rather wait and see what happens or use 'natural remedies', such as vitamins. Drugs are powerful chemicals and they can and do have adverse effects. But they are also the best way to control fits completely and this is very important for your son now and in the future. Your doctor may well understand your fears so don't hesitate to mention them. Talking to other mothers can also help.

Can side-effects be predicted?

Up to a point they can be. All epilepsy drugs have side-effects in common (drowsiness, etc.). Others are known to produce specific side-effects but only in some people (see list on page 57). Although not everyone will get them, it's a good idea for patients to know about these so that they can alert their doctor if they happen. Unfortunately some doctors don't believe in telling their patients about side-effects because they think they will be worried or even imagine them!

Should my drug be changed because I am getting side-effects?

It may or may not be a good idea to do this. If your attacks are completely controlled and the side-effects are not too bad, then staying with this drug may be the best course of action. But only you can judge how bad the side-effects are. Unfortunately changing to another drug may not get rid of the side-effects completely and the control of the fits may not be as good.

If you are experiencing side-effects and are still having fits, then clearly the right treatment for you has not been found.

Will the effects of my drug wear off?
Initial side-effects like drowsiness can wear off or may be helped by a reduction in dose, even if this is increased again at a later date. If a drug controls the fits initially, this control does not usually wear off, and if the fits return, this is usually for another reason (such as forgetting to take the medicine). The only real exception to this is when the group of drugs known as *benzodiazepines* are used to treat the epilepsy. They are usually only used for severe cases. The beneficial effect of these drugs often wears off in time, leading to a return of the fits.

My doctor doesn't seem very interested in the side-effects that I am getting. What can I do?
The main point of drug treatment is to control the fits completely. That's probably why you went to see the doctor in the first place. The fact that you are getting side-effects from otherwise successful treatment may unfortunately seem to be an incidental problem to your doctor. There is also a limited amount that can be done about side-effects without changing your treatment completely which you both may be reluctant to do. Your doctor should be able to explain the options open to you.

Phenytoin

A lot of people do very well on phenytoin, which has been used to treat seizures for many years. However, it can produce side-effects which you should know about and watch out for. If side-effects which trouble you do occur, let your doctor know.

I am taking phenytoin. Why do I need to have blood tests?
Blood tests for levels of anti-epileptic drugs give an indication of the level of the drug in your body, including in your brain, where the drugs work.

There are three main reasons why blood tests for drug levels are needed with phenytoin:

1 If you have too little phenytoin in your blood, it is unlikely to work properly because the level in your brain will also be too low.
2 It is important that you do not have too much of the drug in your body. This can cause side-effects. Your doctor will want to check on the level from time to time.
3 Phenytoin is handled by the body in a slightly different way from other drugs. This means that small changes in the dose you are taking can lead to large changes in the level in your blood. So if your dose is being altered, your doctor will probably want to check your blood levels from time to time.

What would happen if my phenytoin level was high?
Every person is different, and you might have no problems if this happened. However, symptoms often occur when the phenytoin level is high. These include dizziness, unsteadiness, slurred speech and headache. If you develop any of these symptoms, contact your doctor.

If my phenytoin level is high, should my dose be reduced?
It depends on whether or not you have symptoms. You are the best test of whether the level of the drug in your blood is too high; the blood test done in the laboratory is only a guide. If you have a high phenytoin level and remain well, you may be one of those people who can tolerate a level which is higher than average. This higher level may also be required to control your fits.

If you have symptoms of toxicity and your level is high, it is usually necessary to reduce the dose. Because phenytoin is broken down quite slowly, it is usually quite safe to stop taking the drug altogether for twenty-four hours and then to start again at a slightly lower dose, perhaps 25 or 50 mg a day less. You may then have to wait to see whether this reduction gets rid of the symptoms, and the blood test may have to be repeated.

Can I take other drugs while I am taking phenytoin?
Yes, you can. But phenytoin does interfere with some other drugs, and the commonest of these is the contraceptive pill. So you need to make sure your doctor knows you are taking phenytoin when prescribing other medicines for you. If you want to take the Pill, you may well need one with a higher dose of oestrogen than normal. You may need 50 micrograms of oestrogen a day or even more. While the dose is being stabilized, you should use other methods of birth control.

My doctor said I might have to take phenytoin for years. Will it cause any damage?
There are some side-effects which can occur in some people with long-term use. Overgrowth of the gums, so-called *gingival hyperplasia*, is one of these. Good care of your teeth and the advice of a dentist are helpful in avoiding this. If the overgrowth is very bad, your dentist may recommend that your gums are cut back. Sometimes excess body hair is a side-effect, and acne can be made worse.

Can I continue to take phenytoin if I get pregnant?
Phenytoin is best avoided in women who want to have children as it can damage the developing baby. The commonest abnormalities are hare lip, cleft palate and heart defects. These cannot as yet be detected before the baby is born.

If you have decided to have a child you should discuss your drug treatment with your doctor well before you get pregnant so that your drugs can be changed if necessary. Once you are pregnant it's really too late to do this.

Does it matter if my treatment is changed from Epanutin capsules to phenytoin tablets?
You may be used to getting your phenytoin as Epanutin capsules (see table on page 55) and be rather worried if you suddenly get generic phenytoin tablets from your pharmacist instead. They are

the same drug but in a different *formulation*. For most people it makes little difference which you take and the government is trying to encourage the wider use of these generic drugs because they are cheaper and for most people just as good. But if you notice any change in how you feel on the new medicine, talk to your pharmacist or doctor.

Carbamazepine

I have two types of fit, and I'm taking carbamazepine. Will it work on both types?
Carbamazepine is effective in treating both partial seizures and generalized seizures. If these are the sorts of seizure you have, then this drug is suitable for you. It's no use for absences.

Do I need blood tests when taking carbamazepine?
There is a connection between the level of carbamazepine in the blood and its effect on fits, so blood tests can help to find the right dose for you. But it's an easier drug for your doctor to prescribe than phenytoin, so blood tests are only sometimes necessary.

What are the side-effects of carbamazepine?
Carbamazepine does not usually cause too many problems. Symptoms such as loss of appetite, nausea and vomiting may occur when the drug is first introduced, but usually pass. Mild skin rashes are sometimes seen, and the drug may have to be stopped for this reason. Quite commonly, carbamazepine reduces the number of white cells in your blood. In almost all cases, this causes no problems whatever.

If the dose of carbamazepine is too high for you, dizziness, blurred vision and unsteadiness may result. A small reduction in the dose may then be required, which will usually get rid of the side-effects within twenty-four hours as carbamazepine is broken down quickly by the body. Some people taking carbamazepine report that their side-effects come and go during the day. This is because carbamazepine is a relatively short-acting drug and the blood level rises and falls in between doses.

What is Tegretol Retard?
It contains the same drug as other forms of Tegretol, namely carbamazepine. However, the formulation is different. Because carbamazepine is broken down quite quickly in the liver, the manufacturers have made this longer-acting version. You need take it only twice a day and some people find that they get fewer side-effects because the blood level doesn't change quite so much during the day.

Can I take the Pill in the normal way with my carbamazepine?
Like phenytoin and phenobarbitone, carbamazepine interferes with the contraceptive pill because it stimulates the Pill's breakdown in the liver. You should take the same precautions as we have mentioned for phenytoin on page 63.

Is carbamazepine safe in pregnancy?
None of the epilepsy drugs is entirely safe and studies have claimed that carbamazepine can cause growth problems in babies as well as physical abnormalities. But by and large UK experts believe that carbamazepine is amongst the safest epilepsy drugs for women in pregnancy.

Sodium valproate

How does sodium valproate work?
The answer to this question is not really known, but it has been suggested that valproate acts on a brain chemical called GABA and decreases the excitability of the brain. It may also directly affect nerve cells.

Can sodium valproate be used against all seizures?
Sodium valproate has the widest range of anti-epileptic activity of all the drugs. It's effective in all forms of generalized seizures, including tonic-clonic, absence and myoclonic fits. It is also good for partial seizures.

Do I need to have blood tests now that I'm on sodium valproate?
Blood levels do not often give useful information with this drug. Only if you take valproate on its own are blood levels at all helpful.

Should I expect side-effects?
In general, most people don't have any problems with sodium valproate. Loss of appetite, sickness and diarrhoea used to be troublesome, and so coated tablets were developed to prevent this from happening.

Weight gain and hair loss are well-recognized side-effects. They can be lessened by reducing the dose, and the hair loss does not lead to to baldness.

Blood tests can show minor changes in the function of the liver but these rarely lead to problems. The most serious adverse effect is liver failure, which is very rare. It is thought to be more likely to occur in young children with severe epilepsy, those with other handicaps and those on other drugs.

Does sodium valproate interfere with the Pill like the other epilepsy drugs?
No, it doesn't. Unlike phenytoin, carbamazepine and phenobarbitone, sodium valproate does not stimulate the liver and so the normal dose of the Pill can be taken quite safely.

Would sodium valproate be harmful if I got pregnant?
Sodium valproate can cause abnormalities in babies, particularly spina bifida. This can be very serious but it can be detected early on in pregnancy using a special blood test and an ultrasound

examination. These should be done early enough so that you can decide whether you want to continue with the pregnancy.

Phenobarbitone and primidone

My doctor wants to change my medicine from phenobarbitone to carbamazepine. Will this be better for me?

Phenobarbitone is the oldest anti-epileptic in use, having been introduced in 1912. It is an effective anti-epileptic drug, and is used in generalized tonic-clonic seizures and sometimes in partial seizures.

However, there are quite a few problems with phenobarbitone, and so it has fallen out of favour. First, the drug stays in the body for a long time. This means that levels of phenobarbitone may gradually rise, leading to side-effects. These side-effects may appear so gradually that they pass unnoticed. This is especially true of the effect of phenobarbitone on mental functioning. Drowsiness and sedation can be a big problem, although sometimes people get used to this effect. In the longer term, changes in mood and behaviour can occur. In adults this is most likely to be depression and loss of interest.

Second, behaviour disturbances can occur in children leading to extreme excitability and restlessness, the so-called *hyperkinetic syndrome*. This usually comes on quite soon after they have started taking the drug.

Third, phenobarbitone is broken down in the body very slowly and this makes it difficult to alter the dose quickly.

For these reasons, doctors now often prefer to use other drugs. But it's important to realize that many people take phenobarbitone without problems, and don't need to change to another drug. There have to be very good reasons for doing this and you should be warned that your fits could come back even if you are put on another drug.

Someone told me that phenobarbitone and primidone are the same drug. Is that true?

Primidone is broken down in the body into phenobarbitone, and in many respects the two drugs are very similar. But before it's changed into phenobarbitone, primidone itself can cause some unpleasant side-effects. These are usually sickness and dizziness. It's also doubtful if primidone is really any more effective than phenobarbitone at controlling seizures in most people.

Is phenobarbitone safe in pregnancy?

Probably it's reasonably safe for the baby but accurate information on this is lacking.

Ethosuximide

What is ethosuximide used for?

This drug is effective in the treatment of absence seizures. Blood tests for serum levels are sometimes helpful, as there is a relationship between serum level of the drug and its effectiveness. Serious side-effects are rare with this drug. If the dose is too high, nausea, loss of appetite, drowsiness and headache sometimes occur. Little is known about its safety in pregnancy.

Is it necessary to take ethosuximide with other epilepsy drugs?

Children who have absences may also be at risk of tonic-clonic seizures. Unfortunately, ethosuximide won't control this type of seizure and so such children may need to take another drug as well. Alternatively, sodium valproate could be used, which controls both absence and tonic-clonic seizures.

The benzodiazepines

Is Valium a good drug for epilepsy?

Valium, or diazepam, is the best-known member of the group of drugs called *benzodiazepines*. Nitrazepam (Mogadon), clonazepam (Rivotril) and clobazam (Frisium) are also benzodiazepines. They are so effective in stopping someone having a fit that diazepam is given by injection as emergency treatment by doctors. Unfortunately their effect tends to wear off if repeated doses are used. This does not always happen but is quite common, so that these drugs are only given on a regular basis to people with epilepsy if all other treatments have failed. Most of the benzodiazepines are also sedatives and people who take them for epilepsy often complain of being sleepy. This can also make their fits worse.

My daughter has myoclonic epilepsy, and the doctor gave her clonazepam. Is it the right drug?
Yes. The main use of this drug is in the treatment of myoclonic jerks, which can also respond to sodium valproate. Clonazepam is sometimes used for complex absence seizures.

Clonazepam seemed to work well for the first few months, but now my daughter's fits are getting worse. Is the drug wearing off?
Most anti-epileptic drugs do not lose their effect when taken for a long time. But this can occasionally happen with clonazepam. Your daughter should carefully record her fits over a period of time, and you should discuss your concerns at your next appointment with the doctor. If it seems that the drug has really lost its effect, your doctor will discuss alterations to the treatment plan with you both.

It's easy to think that drugs are losing their effect when seizures get worse. This is not usually the case. Epilepsy is a condition which has ups and downs for most people – sometimes seizures improve, and sometimes they are worse. It is often difficult to know why.

My doctor wants me to try clobazam. Will it work?
Clobazam, also called Frisium, has been used quite a lot in people whose seizures are difficult to control. It can be effective, perhaps

particularly with partial seizures. Unlike with the other benzodiazepines, people who have taken this drug often report that it
doesn't make them sleepy. But, as with all drugs in this group, the
effectiveness does tend to wear off with time, something we call
tolerance.

Getting the dose right

Most people are prescribed a single drug initially. This drug is
chosen taking into account the type of attack, the age and sex of the
person, and other factors, such as the doctor's own experience of
treating other patients with a similar problem.

However, although a lot is known about epilepsy and its treatment, there is still an element of trial and error in trying to find the
right drug and the right dose for you. So quite often the starting
dose has to be changed and sometimes other drugs have to be tried.
All this takes time and if more attacks occur, it can give the
impression that treatment is not going to work. But it's very important to stick to a treatment plan and try to control the attacks as
quickly as possible.

*I had another fit just after starting this medicine. Does that mean it's not
going to work?*
No, not necessarily. Drugs take time to build up in the body and the
fit may have occurred before the drug had a chance to work. Also,
the starting dose may not be high enough for you.

*I haven't had an attack since starting these tablets. When can I stop taking
them?*
Your doctor will probably have discussed this with you already,
before you started the treatment. Most doctors advise at least two
years of treatment before thinking about stopping the medicine. In
some young children this period can be shorter. This is discussed
further in Chapter 8 (pages 92–4).

I didn't take my tablets for a week and didn't have another fit. Does this mean the epilepsy has gone away?
Probably not. Some drugs come out of the body quite slowly and so during part of that week you still had the medicine inside you. Also fits do not always occur the moment the drug is stopped.

I don't want my son to take any treatment. Can I stop it?
It's very dangerous to stop taking epilepsy treatment suddenly. This can result in a series of fits called status epilepticus which can be fatal (see page 52). If you have decided not to give your son treatment you should talk it over with your doctor first. Treatment should always be reduced slowly but if he is on no treatment he will be at risk from more fits.

My daughter doesn't want to take her medicine at school. Will she have to?
With the modern treatments most children need only take medicine once or twice a day, so a lunch-time dose should not usually be necessary. If it is, then it's wise to talk to the school as some teachers are not keen on supervising children taking medication. You will also have to think of how other children may react to your daughter taking medicine. Some children with epilepsy have been called 'junkies' by their classmates. So it needs quite a lot of thought and your daughter will need to feel confident about dealing with any difficulties.

I know another child whose fits were controlled on a much smaller dose. Why does my son have to take such a big dose?
The right dose for your son is the dose that controls his attacks without producing intolerable side effects. He is a different person from the other child that you know with a different body metabolism. So he may well require a bigger dose merely for the drug to have the same effect. It doesn't mean that your son's epilepsy is worse than the other child's.

How do you know that I'm on the right dose of the right drug?
Normally patients are started on a low dose of one drug and the dose is not increased unless more fits occur. This way the dose prescribed is likely to be the lowest that will control the attacks. If the first drug chosen controls the attacks without producing unpleasant side-effects, then this is probably the right drug for this person. If serious side-effects occur whether or not the fits are controlled, then another drug is usually tried.

If the fits continue, then the dose of the first drug is usually increased until either the attacks stop or side-effects occur. Blood tests which measure the amount of the drug in the blood can help the doctor decide on the right dose for you. If you still have attacks despite a full dose of one drug, then you may be advised to try another drug instead, going through the same process of building up the dose gradually. The diagram opposite shows the steps that your doctor may follow.

I had another fit and was taken to casualty. The doctor there wanted to change my treatment. Is this right?
While your treatment is being stabilized, it's much better to stick to a treatment plan which should be supervised by one doctor. Un-planned changes to dose or, even worse, another doctor changing your drug just because you had another attack is a thoroughly bad idea. You or the casualty doctor should consult with the doctor who is managing your case. Unfortunately you may not be very popular in casualty if you refuse to change your treatment, so be tactful!

Can I experiment with the dosage of my drug?
It's better not to do this unless your doctor says you can. Some of the epilepsy drugs are rather slow acting and therefore changes in dose may not become fully effective for some days, even weeks. When changing the dose of a drug, it's usually best to make one small change at a time and to allow enough time to monitor the full effect of the change before making another one.

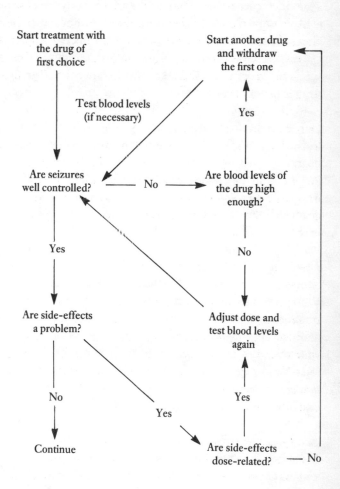

Starting epilepsy treatment

Now that my fits are controlled, the hospital wants my GP to supervise my treatment. Is this a good idea?

It may be very much more convenient for you to see your GP than go to the hospital. Some GPs are taking a lot of interest in managing epilepsy. Your GP can offer continuity which is often difficult in the hospital where you may see a junior doctor rather than the consultant. Both you and your GP may, however, prefer for you to be seen by the consultant again if any problems arise and when you are considering stopping your treatment.

I had another fit after a long time without one. Does my treatment need changing?

Possibly, but not necessarily. It's a good idea to try to identify if anything caused you to have another attack after a period of good control. Missing tablets is a common cause although you may be reluctant to admit this – you may not even realize it has happened. This is by no means the only cause, however, and severe stress or a long period without sleep can do the same thing. Sometimes there is no obvious explanation. Your treatment should certainly be reviewed by the doctor looking after your epilepsy.

Can the doctor tell if I have not been taking my medicine?

It is much better to be open about it if you haven't been taking the treatment as prescribed. You may have a very good reason for this. And it's very difficult to remember to take medicine when you are feeling perfectly well. Measuring the amount of drug in your blood can detect what is called *non-compliance* with treatment. Unfortunately missing doses is not the only reason for low blood levels and patients are sometimes accused quite unjustifiably of not taking their treatment reliably.

I'm not happy with my treatment. How do I get another opinion?

The same principles apply here that we discussed in the context of getting a second opinion about the diagnosis (see page 20). It's important to identify why you are unhappy and what you hope to get out of another opinion. It's also essential that you get the right opinion and that the person you see has all the information about you. Otherwise it can be a great waste of time.

If I see a consultant privately, will I get better treatment?
All the drugs and all the tests that you could need are available under the NHS. So seeing someone privately will not make other treatments available to you. However, paying for advice may mean you can see the person of your choice who may also have more time to devote to you. Your GP is the best person to advise you.

I want my daughter to see a top epilepsy specialist. How can I find one?
All paediatricians and neurologists have a full knowledge of the best way to manage epilepsy. But there are a few specialists in the UK who spend a lot of their time managing the rather more difficult cases. Your GP should be able to refer you to one of these doctors if needed, and you can get further guidance from one of the voluntary organizations (see pages 144–5).

Points to remember

- It takes time for a drug to work fully.
- All epilepsy drugs produce side-effects. These can be minimized by keeping the dose as low as possible and building up the dose slowly and only if more fits occur.
- The newer epilepsy drugs have fewer long-term side-effects.
- Most drugs can be taken once or twice a day.
- A fit occurring after a long period of good control warrants a review of the treatment.
- Avoid casual changes to treatment.
- Different anti-epileptic drugs are used for different seizures.
- Blood tests to find the level of the drug are useful with some drugs but not all.

- Drug treatment is a very individual matter, so it may take time to find what suits you best.
- If you are unhappy with your drug treatment, discuss it fully with your doctor.

For more information about:

– Changing your treatment, see pages 85–9.
– Other types of treatment, see pages 89–91.
– Stopping treatment, see pages 92–4.
– Drugs and pregnancy, see pages 102–4.
– Drugs and schooling, see page 125.

7 My fits haven't stopped yet

As we said in Chapter 3, in about seven out of ten people fits will stop, usually with simple drug treatment. But this leaves three out of ten, or about 100,000 people in the UK, who will continue to have attacks despite appropriate initial treatment.

Quite a lot more more can be done to help people in both categories by fine-tuning their treatment, and also by helping them to control their own attacks.

In this chapter we consider some of the important aspects of treating epilepsy which is initially proving difficult to control.

. . . .

How you can help yourself and your doctor

Although drug treatment is the most reliable way of controlling fits completely, people who continue to have fits can do a lot both to minimize the chances of having them and the effect they have on their daily lives.

Should I keep a record of all my attacks? Will this help the doctor?
It could do, yes. Usually in the first few months after starting epilepsy, it's a good idea to keep a note of when fits have happened as this may help your doctor alter your treatment. Once treatment is stabilized, you should discuss with your doctor whether keeping a record is a good idea and what information is required. The voluntary organizations produce very good diaries for this purpose (see

Date	'Major'	'Minor'	Comments	Month
1				JUNE
2			PERIOD STARTED	
3				
4		XXX		
5				
6			PERIOD OVER	
7				
8				
9				
10				
11		X		
12		XX		
13				
14				
15				
16				
17				
18				
19		XX		
20				
21			EPILIM INCREASED	
22				
23				
24				
25				
26				
27				
28				
29				
30				
31				

Daytime		8	Treatment 1	EPILIM 1500
Sleep		0	2	
Total		8	3	

Page from a fit diary

page 78). It probably isn't a good idea, however, to become too obsessed with noting every detail of all your attacks.

Should I wear a bracelet saying I have epilepsy?
Quite a lot of people with epilepsy recommend this as it helps them get the right assistance if they have a fit. You can have a bracelet inscribed with the diagnosis, an identifying serial number and an emergency phone number. These bracelets can be bought from Medic-Alert and your doctor will be asked to provide some information about you. The SOS Talisman is a necklace or bracelet which contains an information strip giving details of your condition and whom to contact in an emergency. The address of the suppliers of both these personal safety aids is on page 150.

Other people just prefer to carry an information card, produced by one of the voluntary organizations, which they carry in a wallet or handbag. One advantage of the bracelet, however, is that people who come to help you may not want to rummage around in your bag or pockets in case they are accused of trying to steal from you.

I've heard that watching TV can bring on fits. Is this true?
There are some children whose fits may be triggered by watching TV because they are what is known as *photosensitive*. The TV produces a light that flashes very rapidly but which is only visible if you get very close to the screen. Photosensitivity can only be shown on an EEG and it isn't a problem for most people. In those affected it can be overcome by not getting too close to the set, adjusting the set by remote control and having the rest of the room well lit. Sodium valproate can also be helpful.

Should I let my daughter go to discos where they use flashing lights? She also likes video games. Are they a problem?
Ordinary coloured disco lights do not usually flash fast enough to cause a problem. Strobe lights can do so, however, although some local authorities have rules about this, limiting the flash frequency.

The most dangerous frequencies are fifteen to sixty flashes per second. By and large going to discos is a good idea for young people but if your daughter is photosensitive and is exposed to a bright flashing light, all she need do is to turn away from the light and cover one eye with her hand until it stops flashing.

Very strong alternating patterns have been shown to have a similar effect to bright flashing lights in people who are photosensitive. Some video games have these and even some curtain materials and wallpapers.

However, even in susceptible people flashing lights and strong patterns are unlikely to cause a convulsion as the exposure has to be intense and quite prolonged.

Absences can be induced by flickering light such as the reflection of the sun off water or if strong sunlight is seen through trees from a fast-moving vehicle. However, the risk of these phenomena to most people with epilepsy is extremely small. It shouldn't just be assumed that if a person has a fit in front of the TV or where there are flashing lights it was necessarily the TV or lights which triggered the fit.

Can stress bring on fits?
Yes, it can. But stress is a part of normal living and can't really be avoided. It's better to find ways of dealing with stressful situations in a way that does not increase your own level of stress. Expert counselling could help you if stress is a major factor for you.

My son always seems to have fits when I ask him to do something he doesn't want to do. How should I handle this?
It isn't easy. No parent wants to cause fits in a child, and the sight of your son having an attack apparently as a result of something that you have done will certainly increase your level of stress. It's tempting to avoid these confrontations and over-indulge children as a result. But this won't help either in the long run. Having a family discussion, including your son, when you are all relaxed and in a

good mood, may sort out the problem but you may also need outside advice.

I didn't drink tea for a week and didn't have any fits. Does this mean that tea causes my attacks?
Although some people are convinced that certain foods or drinks trigger their fits, overall this is hard to prove. If you find that some foods regularly upset you, then it's sensible to avoid them. But it's equally important to eat a balanced diet and, for social reasons, not to have too many restrictions on what you eat.

One doctor I saw said I shouldn't drink alcohol. Must I stop?
This rather depends on your drinking habits and whether you think it affects the control of your fits. Alcohol can induce fits in some people who do not have epilepsy. These are actually alcohol with-drawal fits and usually occur after a binge. So potentially large amounts of alcohol could trigger your fits, but modest amounts are unlikely to do you much harm. Drinking is important to some people's social life, and no one would want you to become a hermit. If going to pubs is important to you but you would rather avoid alcohol, it's quite acceptable to drink low- or no-alcohol drinks which are widely available now. A lot of people prefer them because they want to keep fit or drive.

It's also possible that the side-effects of your drugs and alcohol could add together. The alcohol could also theoretically speed up the metabolism of the drugs by your liver, thus making your drugs less effective. But most people don't report a problem.

A high temperature always brings on my daughter's fits. What can I do about it?
It's known that fever (raised body temperature) can bring on fits in some very young children, so-called febrile convulsions (see page 43). Most of these children don't go on to develop epilepsy. As children get older this tendency wears off, but some parents notice

that a fever often brings on fits in their child who has epilepsy. Sometimes, however, it's not in fact a fever that is bringing on the fits, but the fits that are making a child hot and sweaty as though the child has a proper fever.

Some parents say that paracetamol and tepid sponging are useful in older children with epilepsy and occasionally a doctor will recommend giving the child antibiotics as soon as an illness starts, in the hope of preventing a fever and fits. But not all doctors agree with this practice.

Sometimes my daughter's fits go on for ages. I find this terrible to watch. What should I do?
Most people feel that they should be doing something when they see a person having a fit. But there isn't much you can do in most circumstances to make the fit stop. However, first aid measures are always important (see pages 26–9).

It is essential that you, as a parent, and other members of your family have the opportunity to discuss what you should do when fits occur. A management plan of when to call for help needs to be agreed with your doctor. The same applies to a husband, wife or partner of an adult with epilepsy. Most fits are quite short, lasting less than a minute, although they may seem to be very long to the person watching. So usually there is no need to do anything apart from applying the normal first aid procedure.

Some children are, however, prone to very long fits or serial attacks (one attack after another with partial recovery in between). If these fits are accompanied by breathing difficulties, the child is in danger of brain damage. Parents can be taught how to give diazepam to stop the fits and the most convenient way to give this is by injection into the rectum, using a special tube (see illustration on page 44). Diazepam given rectally can also be useful for stopping prolonged seizures in adults. The dose to be given will be decided by your doctor.

My fits are always worse at the time of my periods. Is this common and what can be done about it?

Yes, it is common, although we don't know exactly what causes it to happen. Ways of preventing it include taking a water pill (a *diuretic*) or increasing the dose of the normal epilepsy medicines before the period starts, taking the contraceptive pill and various forms of progesterone therapy. Doctors sometimes prescribe clobazam (Frisium) to be taken just before the period starts and for the first few days of the period. None of these treatments is effective in all women but they can be worth a try under medical supervision.

Removal of the womb (*hysterectomy*) is not advised as a way of treating menstrually related fits and should only be carried out for gynaecological reasons.

My son goes out until late at night and I'm sure this brings on his fits. How can I make him see sense?

Certainly going without sleep for long periods can induce fits in some people and indeed this is used to provoke attacks when special EEG tests are being carried out. The odd late night isn't going to do any harm and as it is a normal part of being young shouldn't be particularly discouraged. If the fits became a regular event after every late night, your son might decide for himself that missing sleep isn't worth it.

I always seem to have a fit on a Thursday. Why does this happen?

The reason is not obvious. Some people report that their fits go in cycles but there isn't much research on this. If you are really sure that you always have an attack on Thursdays, it's worth examining what you do on Wednesdays to see if there could be anything that triggers your attacks.

Points to remember

- Flashing lights only cause problems to a minority of people and can be easily avoided.
- Stress can trigger fits but stress cannot be avoided in life. Ways of dealing with it have to be found.
- Some people are sure that certain foods bring on their attacks but changes to diet will not help in most cases.
- Alcohol in moderation should not cause problems.
- Most fits are quite short and do not need any medical treatment. But relatives can give rectal diazepam if fits are prolonged.
- Fits are commonly worse at the time of menstruation.
- Long periods without sleep may bring on attacks.

For more information about:

– EEGs, see page 85.
– Life-styles, see Chapter 9 (pages 107–29).
– Emergency treatment, see pages 109–10.

Special tests

Are there any special tests which would help my treatment?
As most people's fits stop quite quickly, the number of those needing special tests is quite small. So these tests are usually carried out at specialized centres. A new scan, the Magnetic Resonance Imaging (MRI) scan gives a very detailed picture of the brain. This type of scan is not widely available: its main role is in situations where detailed information about brain structure is needed – such as when surgery is planned, or when a doctor very strongly suspects that there may be a tumour which has not been shown by other more readily available tests, such as a CT scan.

Would another EEG help get my treatment right?
A special type of EEG test called *EEG monitoring* might give useful information. This is a special form of the EEG (see pages 12–13) which allows the person to go about normal activities while having an EEG recorded. This can go on for several hours or even days.

There are essentially two ways people may be monitored. In both systems electrodes are fixed to the scalp in the usual way. In the system called *ambulatory monitoring* the electrodes feed into a portable cassette recorder which is carried by the person (see page 86). The cassette tape is removed and analysed later. The other system is called *EEG telemetry.* Here the electrical impulses from the electrode are beamed by radio waves to a distant recorder, or, more simply, via a long length of wire, and the EEG trace can be read immediately. Often with this system the person's activity is also recorded by a camera on to videotape.

The purpose of monitoring is often to record an actual fit while the EEG is being recorded. Monitoring is only used in special situations, for example when the diagnosis of epilepsy is doubted or the type of seizure is not clear, if the seizures have not responded to treatment, or if surgery is being considered and the doctors want to know exactly where in the brain the fit starts.

How the drugs can help

Why have I had a fit now, after a year without any?
There is no simple answer to this question. Seizures sometimes occur because the blood level of the drug has fallen. A number of other things – such as alcohol, tiredness, stress – may bring on a fit, but generally we can't say why you have had a seizure at any particular time.

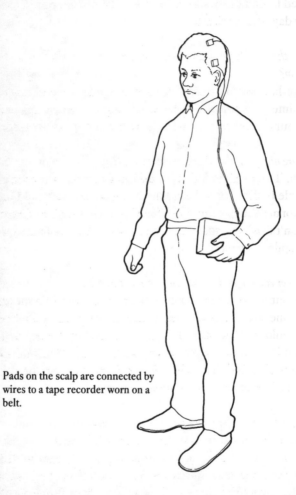

Pads on the scalp are connected by wires to a tape recorder worn on a belt.

Continuous EEG monitoring

Should I take extra medicine if I have more attacks?
No, this is not the best way to control fits completely. You and your
doctor need to find the best regular treatment which you will have to
take every day as prescribed.

*I've been on three different doses of this drug and I'm still having fits. What
happens now?*
If you have had a good trial of a particular drug – which means a
period of time on a dose which is high enough – and are still having
seizures, your doctor will probably wish to try you on a different drug.

If I take more of my present drug, will that help?
It could do. The maximum dose of drug is a very individual matter.
Some people both need and can tolerate a dose which would be far
too much for another person. Everybody's metabolism is different, so
you shouldn't think that just because you need a higher than average
dose your epilepsy is more severe.

Will I be better controlled if I take more than one drug?
About one out of every ten people gets better fit control if they take
more than one drug. But such combination treatment, called polytherapy, should only be started if all the drugs have been tried on
their own. It is often necessary to increase the dose of the individual
drugs until intolerable side-effects occur. Only then can the doctor
know that this particular drug is not going to work.

Which drugs in combination will give the best fit control?
This is a very individual matter. Provided that you have been seeing
the same doctor throughout it should be reasonably easy to decide
which of your drugs have given the best control in the past, and
normally these would be chosen to be taken together. Problems often
arise, however, if you have changed your doctor and some of the
information about the effectiveness of the previous drugs is missing.

Will taking more than one drug give me more side-effects?
Yes, probably it will. Unfortunately drug side-effects don't usually cancel each other out, but tend to add together.

How will I know which of the drugs I am taking is the one that is helping me, and which is the one which is giving me side-effects?
It's very difficult to know this once polytherapy has been started. You can only find out by trial and error, by reducing or increasing the dose of your drugs, under your doctor's supervision, to see what happens. But only make one change at a time and wait long enough for the full effect of the change to be effective.

When I have tried a new drug in the past, it seemed to work for a while and then I got more fits again. Why is this?
People whose fits are proving difficult to control often say this. The hope that a new drug may work can be a powerful form of treatment in its own right but if the drug is not tackling the underlying problem then the fits will inevitably return.

Adding a second drug hasn't helped me. Should I go back to one drug or add a third?
Adding more drugs is a law of diminishing returns. The chances of a third drug helping your fits is very small, but the risk of more side-effects is large. If adding a second drug has not helped you at all, it is sensible for most people to return to single drug therapy (monotherapy).

Will altering the dose of my drugs on days when I feel I may have a fit help to control them?
Most of the epilepsy drugs are quite slow-acting, and therefore increasing the dose today won't have much effect, good or bad, for several days. Some people find adjusting their dose helpful, for example just before menstruating when they are prone to more fits.

Is there anything I can do to make absolutely sure I don't have an attack on an important occasion, for example during an exam or when I get married?
Nothing can be guaranteed to work and you may be even more likely to have an attack if you are very uptight about it (see page 90). For some people, taking a small extra dose of medicine could be helpful or a small dose of a short-acting drug like diazepam or clobazam. Your doctor should be able to advise you. But you should experiment with this several times first. You don't want to fall asleep during the wedding ceremony!

Why do I have to continue to take drugs at all if I am still having fits? Can't I stop the medicine to see what happens?
Well, you could, but you would probably find that the frequency and severity of your attacks would get a lot worse. There's also the danger of status epilepticus (see page 52). This could be very serious. But if you are really determined to reduce your medicine, you need your doctor's advice and support. Any reductions in treatment should be small and gradual.

Non-drug treatments

Would homoeopathy help?
Probably not, but there is no harm in trying. Homoeopathic remedies can be prescribed under the NHS and you should tell the homoeopathic practitioner all about your epilepsy and the treatment you take for it. Other forms of alternative medicine (herbal remedies, acupuncture, etc.) can be tried, although they are not all available on the NHS. Your conventional drugs should not be changed while you are trying out these new treatments until you and your doctor are sure that these new treatments are really working. This could require some months or years to be sure.

Would an operation help me?
It could if you have the right sort of epilepsy and drug treatment

hasn't controlled the fits completely. Knowing whether you would be suitable can involve a lot of tests in most cases. It has to be shown that only a small part of your brain is responsible for your fits. This part of your brain must be in an area which can be removed safely without causing a lot of damage to other brain functions. So not very many people can be helped by an operation. But for those who can, it may cure the epilepsy.

What sorts of operation are commonly done?
The most common type of seizure treated by surgery are complex partial seizures which begin in the temporal lobe. The operation is called *temporal lobectomy* and involves removing the smallest amount of brain tissue possible. Tests are used to pinpoint precisely the area where the seizures are starting. Two other forms of epilepsy surgery are discussed on page 109.

How do I get the tests that I need to see if I'm suitable for an operation?
You need to talk this over with the doctor who is managing your epilepsy, and you may need to be referred to a consultant neuro-logist if you are not already seeing one. Surgery should be con-sidered in all patients who have not responded to drug treatment but unfortunately there are very few centres in the UK which specialize in epilepsy surgery, and comparatively few operations are carried out in the UK each year. You may well find that you have to wait quite a time before the necessary tests can be carried out. The voluntary organizations may be able to tell you more about where surgery for epilepsy is being done.

Would relaxation therapy help me?
We could all probably benefit from learning how to relax properly, particularly when stressed. Techniques such as relaxation or yoga could well help you cope with the day-to-day stresses of life. This may then have an influence on the frequency of your seizures. However, it is unlikely that this sort of therapy would stop your fits

altogether as we still don't really know why they happen when they do.

I've heard that something called biofeedback *helps some people. What is it?*

This is a technique which people can learn which helps them to control their own EEG patterns. Unfortunately it's difficult to do and requires a lot of equipment and training. There is also no real evidence yet that the good effects last for very long. It's best regarded as experimental.

Points to remember

- Taking two drugs instead of one does not always improve fit-control and may increase side-effects.
- Short-term changes to drug dosage do not often improve fit control but may help confidence.
- Even if the fits continue, the drugs are probably still reducing their frequency and severity.
- Alternative remedies could help some people but regular medicines should be continued.
- An operation on the brain can cure the epilepsy in the minority of people who are suitable for this treatment.

For more information about:

Drugs, their uses and side-effects

Epilepsy: prejudice and fact by Mogens Dam and Lennart Gram. Published by Munksgaard (paperback for patients)

A Textbook of Epilepsy (3rd edition) edited by Laidlaw, Richens and Oxley. Chapter on clinical pharmacology and medical treatment by Beth Rimmer and Alan Richens. Published by Churchill Livingstone (hardback textbook for doctors)

8   My fits are now controlled

For the seven out of ten people whose fits stop quite quickly, usually with treatment, epilepsy should, in theory, be only a temporary problem. Unfortunately, in the experience of many, this is not the case, usually because of other people's ignorance of the facts.

In this chapter we look at some of the on-going difficulties that you may face even though your attacks are now completely controlled. This may affect getting a job, driving and having children. Inevitably, once the fits are controlled, many people first of all want to think about stopping their treatment.

.   .   .   .

Stopping treatment

Do I need to stay on a drug for the rest of my life?
This very much depends on the details of your particular experience. Most doctors would want their patient to be completely free of seizures for at least two years before considering stopping drugs. There is a risk of further seizures when drugs are withdrawn, so this needs to be considered carefully. You and your doctor need to weigh up the risks and benefits together before starting to withdraw tablets.

I've not had a fit for three years. How likely am I to have one if I stop my drug?
There is always a risk of seizures returning, and this risk can be difficult to predict for the individual. Studies in recent years with

people stopping anti-epileptic drugs have shown a lot of different results. The number of people who have seizures again is called the *relapse rate* and this has varied from fifteen in 100 people to as high as seven in ten. However, some people are less likely to have problems. In particular, people who have only ever had a few attacks, whose epilepsy has been quickly controlled by treatment, and who have generalized, rather than partial or mixed, seizures (see pages 45–51) are the most likely to be able to stop their medicine without further problems.

Return of seizures is most likely to occur during the period of withdrawal of medication, which should be done slowly and under careful medical supervision.

Can doctors guarantee that my daughter will never have another fit, even if she continues to take medication?
No, they can't. But once your daughter has been free of fits for two years, it is thought that the risk of further attacks would be small enough for her to be allowed to drive a car, if she were old enough. But even people who continue to take medication sometimes have more fits after a long period of good control.

My daughter will leave school in two years' time. Should she stop her medicine now?
By and large it is felt to be a good thing to try to stop her treatment before she leaves school and in many cases this is possible, but not in all. There is always the risk that the fits will return. So this isn't an easy decision and you and your daughter need to think about it very carefully before deciding what to do. Your daughter's doctor will advise you on the basis of the facts of her case.

Before deciding, it's vital that you are sure that she is really completely free of all attacks and free of all other events associated with epilepsy, for example, auras and jerks. If you are in any doubt, discuss it with your daughter's doctor.

Wouldn't it be better to wait until she's a bit older and the fits have been controlled for longer?

The reason for trying to stop her medicine at this time, is that it gets progressively more difficult to take this decision as the young person gets older. A young adult has more to lose than a child – for example, a driving licence – if the fits return.

Can't my daughter have an EEG to see if she can come off medication?

Unfortunately the EEG is not reliable in this situation, but often another recording will be done. If it shows a lot of activity associated with epilepsy, then the doctor will probably advise that your daughter remains on treatment. Even if the EEG is completely normal, this is not a guarantee that the fits won't return.

If she stops treatment and the fits come back, does she go back on to the same medicine?

This is probably what the doctor would advise, but not necessarily. Before starting to discontinue the medicine, which can be a slow process, your doctor needs to tell you what to do if your daughter has another attack. There are a number of options. It is sometimes right just to see what happens next and not to increase the medicine again. In other situations only the last reduction in dose should be restored and in others the full dose should be taken again.

If the fits come back will the treatment be effective again?

Usually it will be but unfortunately not always. For a while it is sometimes necessary to use a higher dose than before to regain control but even this is not successful in every case. We do not fully understand why this should be so but it is possible that the return of the fits disturbs the brain in such a way that the drugs have a much more difficult task in future.

Working

Now that my fits are fully controlled, do I need to tell anyone about what happened in the past?
In most situations it's your choice whether you tell them or not. Often it won't be important to do so but sometimes you have to. If you apply for a driving licence or any form of life or health insurance you'll have to make a declaration. But read the wording of any form carefully. For example, it may not be necessary to declare epilepsy if you are applying for a job unless it is covered by a health regulation. But it's essential that any doctor or other health professional you consult knows that you have a history of fits.

When I put details about my epilepsy on a job application form, I don't get an interview. Should I lie about my epilepsy?
Application forms are often screened by non-medically trained staff who may simply reject anyone who has had any kind of health problem. You certainly mustn't lie on the form, but some people with epilepsy recommend that you leave this part of the form blank. You must, however, then tell the person interviewing you about your epilepsy. But choose your moment and sell yourself first.

I have applied unsuccessfully for several jobs. Am I being discriminated against?
Yes, possibly, but not necessarily. If you're in a very competitive field you may not have the same qualifications or experience as other applicants or you may just have been unlucky. Employers have an absolute right to decide whom they employ and do not have to give a reason for not taking you on. Under UK law, they can discriminate against you because of your epilepsy if they want to, although few would admit to doing this.

Not many jobs are barred by law to people who have controlled epilepsy. More details are given in the list on page 96. Unfortunately some employers, knowing little about epilepsy, assume that you will inevitably have more attacks and that this is bound to cause safety problems at work and trouble with other staff members.

Problem jobs for people with epilepsy

Absolute bar if fits have ever occurred

London underground train driver and track worker

Absolute bar if fits have occurred since fifth birthday

Ambulance crew
Armed Services
Commercial aircraft pilot
Diver
Fire brigade officer
Heavy goods vehicle driver (lorries)
Merchant seaman
Public service vehicle driver (buses)
Taxi driver
Train driver

Health regulations may apply if fits have occurred after the age of five

Care assistant
Commercial driver
Nurse
Police
Teacher in State school
Worker in construction and heavy industry

Health regulations may apply if fits are not controlled

Many

It's worth looking at how you put over the fact that you have epilepsy to employers to make sure that you're not inadvertently putting them off. Do you have to put it on the application form and if so are you doing this in a way that the employer would find reassuring or worrying? If you get to an interview, can you explain about the epilepsy in simple terms? Choosing the right moment to mention your epilepsy is very important. People with epilepsy who have been successful in getting jobs often say that they sell themselves as a person and as a valuable employee first and only mention the epilepsy when they think they have been successful.

Most job interviewers will know almost nothing about epilepsy and so it's a good idea to have a few clear facts about epilepsy at your fingertips and then to give brief details about the way that it affects you personally. Needless to say, looking and sounding confident helps a great deal. Having a letter from your doctor supporting what you say may also help.

Where can I get information about the health requirements of different jobs?
If you are still at school, the school careers advisory service should be able to tell you. If you have left school, you could contact:

- the relevant trade or professional association
- the Employment Medical Advisory service (via your local branch of the Health and Safety Executive)
- your local Job Centre
- the voluntary organizations

If you want to be sure of a good reception from an employer, you could look for the new symbol, launched in 1990 by the government. Employers can use this symbol if they adhere to the Code of Good Practice for the employment of disabled people which was published in 1984 (see page 98).

Sympathetic employer's symbol

I still want to do one of the jobs you say are barred to people with epilepsy. Can I still apply?
You can, but if the job you are going for is controlled by a law or health regulations and you are ineligible, then you will inevitably fail. You may find this demoralizing. It's a good idea to find out as much as you can about the health requirements of your intended trade or profession before you set your sights on a particular job. You may find that you know more about the health requirements than the person interviewing you!

My employer has been fine about my epilepsy but I am not getting promoted. Is this because of the epilepsy?
It's very unlikely to be the reason unless promotion would make some extra demands on you that your employer thinks might be a problem. Have you asked your employer why you have not been promoted? If you have, but without getting a satisfactory answer, someone else, such as your doctor, could ask on your behalf.

Driving

How do I get a driving licence now that my fits have stopped?
If you haven't driven before, fill in the ordinary driving licence application form, answering all the questions including the one which asks about fits, etc. If you enter some details here about your medical history, you will be sent another form by the Driving and Vehicle Licensing Centre (DVLC) asking when your last attack

was. It will also request the name of your doctor who will be asked to confirm the details of your case.

In order to be able to hold a licence, you must have been free from all attacks and other events associated with epilepsy, including auras and jerks, for two years. Any of these events, however minor and whatever the circumstances, occurring during this period will disqualify you. This applies even if you had a very minor attack directly as a result of a change of treatment advised by your doctor.

The only exception to the two-year rule is if you only have attacks while asleep. In this case, you can get a licence despite having attacks, provided that they only occur while you are asleep and provided that at least three years have elapsed from the date of your first fit to the date from which the licence is to be effective, during which time you have only had sleep attacks. All the criteria for holding a licence are subject to the proviso that you are not likely to be a danger to the public for any reason.

Once you have got your provisional licence you still have to pass the driving test. Once you have done this the issue of a full licence is usually subject to a periodic review, which will request up-to-date confirmation that you are still fit-free.

If you have held a driving licence before, you should complete the normal application form, giving your licence number.

I have only ever had fits while asleep but the DVLC say I can't drive again until three years have passed since my fits first started. Why is this?
Quite a lot of people who start by having sleep fits go on to have one while awake. Obviously if you were driving at the time this might be disastrous. So if you continue to have attacks while asleep, the DVLC require a three-year period to elapse from the time your first sleep fit happened before you will be allowed to drive again. This helps to ensure that you are not one of the people who will have an attack while awake. Of course, if your attacks started as sleep fits and then stop altogether, you will be allowed to hold a licence after only two years.

I had a few fits while awake but the last one of these was just over two years ago. I got my licence back recently but my wife said that I had an attack while asleep last week. Can I still drive?

No, you can't. Although you haven't had a fit while awake in the last two years, you've had one while asleep, and there hasn't been a period of three years during which you have only had fits while asleep.

Does my son have to come off his tablets in order to drive?

No. He doesn't. The law does not distinguish between people with controlled epilepsy who are still on drugs and those who have stopped their medication. It is the complete control of the attacks that is the crucial issue. Doctors usually recommend that a person does not drive if their medicine is being reduced for a period of at least six months after the reduction is over. This is because reducing treatment can sometimes trigger another fit.

Will my seventeen-year-old son have to pay more for car insurance?

As a seventeen-year-old he will probably find that his insurance premiums are quite high anyway. But because he is driving quite legally, the fact that he had some fits several years ago should not count against him. If he has difficulty getting cover, it would be advisable to contact one of the voluntary epilepsy associations.

My son has always wanted to earn his living by driving. Can he do this?

It has always been official medical policy that people who have had fits, even if they are now completely controlled, should not be encouraged to drive for a living. The law prohibits anyone from holding a Heavy Goods Vehicle (HGV) or Public Service Vehicle (PSV) licence if that person has ever had a fit since reaching the age of five years. The same rule applies to taxi drivers who are licensed by a local authority. There is no actual law in the UK regarding other forms of driving for a living (such as commercial traveller, van driver, etc.) which do not require a special licence. But if an employer asks for a medical opinion about your son's suitability for such a job, the doctor will usually advise against it. The reason for this is that statistically your son is still more likely to have another fit than the next person, even if his fits are now completely controlled. So it is felt that someone like your son should not be encouraged to spend a lot of time driving as this increases the chance of having a fit at the wheel.

I had some jerking movements just after waking up. What are they and can I go on driving?
Probably they are myoclonic jerks (sudden twitching of the arms, legs or body). They count as fits and you should stop driving immediately and inform the DVLC. You won't be allowed to drive again for two years even if you never have any more.

My fits stopped some years ago and I now drive a car. My doctor wants me to reduce my tablets. Should I do this?
This is a difficult decision and needs a lot of thought. If you have another attack, even if it's only an aura or a jerk as a result of reducing your treatment on medical advice, you will still lose your licence. You will only get it back when you have again been free of fits for two years. The same rule applies if you have another attack as a result of being ill, forgetting to take your medicine or because of someone else's mistake, such as a doctor prescribing the wrong tablets or a pharmacist's mistake in dispensing them. So before reducing your medicine you need to consider how valuable your driving licence is to you.

I hold a UK driving licence but can I drive abroad?
In EC countries the UK driving licence is valid for up to one year if you are just visiting. If you intend staying longer you will need a licence issued by the country concerned and their rules about epilepsy will apply. If you intend driving in other countries you may need an International Driving Licence. For further information contact the DVLC Drivers' Enquiry Unit in Swansea.

I know I can't drive on the road because I'm still having fits. But can I drive on private property?

Yes, you can. But you must be very careful not to go anywhere which is a public highway or where members of the public are likely to be driving. You are still putting yourself at risk by driving when your fits are not fully controlled. It's also most unlikely that you will get any insurance cover.

Some people ask this question because they need to drive a vehicle such as fork lift truck while they are at work. So long as they only drive on an employer's private premises, a driving licence is not required. But if an employer asks for a medical opinion whether this is safe, most doctors would say that the two-year free of fits rule should be applied.

Having a baby

My husband and I want to start a family. Should I stop taking my medicine?

The decision whether to continue to take treatment or not is usually made independently of your wanting to become pregnant. However, many women are concerned that the drugs they take may harm their baby and for this reason alone want to stop treatment. Unfortunately, none of the epilepsy drugs is entirely safe in pregnancy, although carbamazepine is generally thought to be the least harmful. It is also important that you take the minimum number of drugs to control your attacks, as the more drugs taken, the bigger the risk to the baby. It's wise to tell your doctor as far in advance as possible of your intention to have a baby so that your treatment can be reassessed. Sometimes patient and doctor will decide that the medicine can be stopped, but this should only be done under medical supervision. You need time to consider all the issues involved and get expert advice.

If I had another fit as a result of stopping the treatment, would I have to start it again while I was pregnant?
Probably this would be advisable as being free of fits during pregnancy is important. Once the pregnancy has lasted for more than three months, the risk to the baby from your medicine is much less.

If I decide to continue to take my treatment, what could happen to my baby?
Probably your baby would be perfectly all right. However, all the epilepsy drugs can cause damage to the developing baby although most of these malformations are relatively minor. The risk of birth deformities in babies whose mothers are being treated for epilepsy is about two to three times greater than usual. Phenytoin is known to cause hare lip and cleft palate in some children, and sodium valproate has been blamed for causing spina bifida. Spina bifida is an abnormality of the base of the spine which can cause severe difficulties with walking and bladder control. This malformation can be detected during early pregnancy using a blood test and an ultrasound examination. The defect cannot be corrected but the woman can decide whether to continue with the pregnancy. Other deformities which are known to occur include congenital heart disease, abnormalities of the skeleton and intestines.

Should my treatment be changed now that I have become pregnant?
It certainly is not worth reducing treatment now that you know that you are pregnant as the baby has already been exposed to your drug during the critical period when the baby's organs are being formed. In this situation, keeping the fits controlled is the main priority. Occasionally it is necessary to increase the dose during the later stages of pregnancy but this is usually only done if more fits occur. Monitoring the blood level of your drug during pregnancy is often an advisable course.

Would it be safer for my baby if I stopped my drugs just before getting pregnant and then started them again later?

It might be, but there isn't much research on this. It could be risky for you as you could have more fits by stopping your drugs. You shouldn't try without your doctor's agreement. You would also need to be free of drugs for some weeks before getting pregnant. And even if you don't take them again for at least three months, there's still no absolute guarantee that the drugs couldn't have a harmful effect on the baby as it grows inside you.

My fits stopped some years ago. Am I likely to have fits again when I am pregnant and will this harm my baby?

A few women only have fits when pregnant due to the various changes that take place in the woman's body. Being free of attacks when pregnant is obviously very important for both mother-to-be and baby but even so, neither is likely to come to much harm if a fit should occur. If the fits start again, however, you should get expert advice quickly.

Can I have my baby normally or will I have to have a caesarean?

You should certainly have your baby in hospital but there is no particular reason why it should not be a normal delivery. Obviously the doctor and midwife must know about the epilepsy.

Will I be able to breast-feed?

Yes, and this is recommended wherever possible. Although the drug you take may well be in your breast milk, this is nothing new to the baby who was exposed to it while inside you. But if the baby feeds poorly and seems to be very sleepy, breast-feeding may have to be stopped.

Can I pass my epilepsy on to my child?

This does happen in some families. But whether you will or not depends on many factors which we do not entirely understand.

Certainly epilepsy does seem to run in some families and any child born to a mother with epilepsy has an increased risk of developing it. The risk to anyone in the general population is about one in 200 and to a child of a mother with epilepsy it may be as high as one in twenty-five. If both parents have epilepsy, particularly if there is no known cause, the risk to the child may be as high as one in four. If you have a family history of epilepsy or are worried about the risk to your child, you should ask to be referred to a genetic counsellor, preferably before the pregnancy starts.

My epilepsy started after I banged my head and there is no one else in my family or my partner's family who has it. Does this mean my baby will not get epilepsy?
There is no simple answer to this question. The answer must be based on information about probabilities. The fact that you are the only person affected in your family means that the risk to your child is less. But even so, statistically speaking, your child still has a greater chance of developing epilepsy than someone in the general population (who has a one in 200 chance). Lots of people bang their heads and don't get epilepsy, so you probably have a tendency to have seizures which you may pass on to your child.

Can my child have a test to see whether epilepsy is present?
No. No test will predict the future. The usual tests (EEGs, etc.) would be carried out if your child's doctor thought that your child might have had a fit, but usually not otherwise.

Should I tell my child about my epilepsy?
This is really for you to decide but it could be important for your child to know. Many mothers with epilepsy recommend that you do tell your children. First, you may still be taking treatment and your child may wonder why. And second, it could be relevant information when he or she is considering starting a family in years to come.

Points to remember

- Many people can stop their treatment successfully after about two years free of attacks.
- Deciding whether to stop treatment needs careful consideration as adults, in particular, often have a lot to lose if the fits return.
- Only a few occupations are barred by law to people who have had fits. Applying for jobs where there are special safety factors may not be successful.
- Epilepsy should be disclosed to an employer, if appropriate, but application forms are often not the best way of doing this.
- People with epilepsy may drive when they have been completely free of attacks for two years, provided they are not a danger to the public for other reasons.
- Jerks and auras count as fits as far as the law on driving is concerned.
- A person who has had any fits since reaching the age of five years may never hold an HGV or PSV licence and other forms of driving for a living are officially discouraged.
- Most mothers with epilepsy have healthy babies. But epilepsy drugs can cause malformations. Reassessment of treatment should take place well before the pregnancy.
- A child born to a mother with epilepsy has an increased risk of developing epilepsy.

For more information about:

Driving

Enquiries about driving can be made direct to Medical Branch, DVLC, Oldway Centre, Swansea SA6 7JL   Tel: 0792 72151.

Working

'Epilepsy', Chapter 12 in *Fitness for Work*, ed. Edwards, McCallum and Taylor (Oxford Medical Publications). Also *Epilepsy and Employment – a medical symposium on current problems and best practices*, ed. Edwards, Espir and Oxley (Royal Society of Medicine, ICSS No. 86).

9   Living with seizures

Most people with epilepsy whose attacks come under control quite quickly will not really need this chapter. But for those who do, access to accurate information may help to reduce the impact that this disability can have. Many of the topics covered in Chapter 7 are relevant here, but in this last chapter we look at some of the special problems that continuing seizures can bring. It is important to realize, however, that not everyone will have these problems and that solutions are often a very individual matter. So even if we often can't give very specific answers we hope that our comments will help these issues to be thought about and discussed.

. . . .

Managing the seizures

How do I know that my fits are not going to stop?
You don't, is the simple answer. Doctors, like everyone else, cannot predict the future with certainty. But they do have information from research about epilepsy which can be used as a guide when talking about your condition. First, if you have had frequent seizures for years, have tried most or all of the anti-epileptic drugs, and surgery has nothing to offer, then it is not very likely that your seizures will come under full control. Second, partial seizures, especially complex partial seizures, tend to be quite difficult to control. In this particular situation a new diagnosis of *epilepsy resistant to current therapy* is appropriate.

It is important not to lose hope, however. Sometimes fits do improve for no clear reason. Research is going on all the time, and there are a lot of new drugs being developed for epilepsy as well as improvements in surgical techniques.

My specialist wants me to try an experimental drug. Should I agree?
Before you decide, you need to weigh up the pros and cons very carefully. Your specialist should allow you plenty of time to decide and give you as much information as you need about the new drug.

If a drug is still at an experimental stage, there is no guarantee that it will ever be marketed by the drug company. So even if it helps you, it may still be withdrawn from use and you will have to stop taking it. You will also be taking a drug which has not yet been tried extensively in other people and so there will be a great deal that doctors still do not know about it. To this extent you are taking a risk in trying it. And fits can also get worse rather than better when treatment is changed.

But your specialist would not advise an experimental drug unless there was a reasonable chance that it would help you. The use of such drugs in so-called *drug trials* is strictly controlled and you will have a lot of safety checks. By taking the drug you will be contributing to what doctors know about the new treatment and helping with progress in research as well as possibly improving your own fit-control.

Would an operation help my son who has very severe and frequent fits?
The most commonly performed operation for epilepsy is total or partial removal of one temporal lobe (see page 90). By this time your son should have been assessed for his suitability for such an operation. If he has very severe epilepsy and possibly other handicaps, then it's unlikely that his fits are coming from one small area of the brain that can be removed safely.

There are two other types of operation that should be considered, however. They both have very long names. One is called *hemispherectomy* and the other is *callosotomy*. People who have a severe weakness down one side of the body, called *hemiplegia*, may have such severe brain damage on the opposite side that removal of the very damaged half of the brain (*hemispherectomy*) will help control their attacks and not produce any more disability.

The other type of operation on the brain, called *callosotomy*, involves the surgeon cutting some of the nerve fibres that join one side of the brain to the other. It has been shown to be helpful in some people who have severe drop attacks, although other types of fit may continue unchanged.

If my fits get a lot worse, should my treatment be changed?
In some situations this can be useful, but we need to remember that by this time you should have tried all the available drugs at maximum tolerated doses and so you should now be on the drug or drugs that have been found to be the most useful for you. So it may not be obvious how your treatment can be improved. It's absolutely vital to avoid casual changes to your treatment based on lack of knowledge of what has been tried before. Some people understandably 'want something to be done' if their fits get worse. Others are content just to wait and see what happens. Often the fits will revert to their previous pattern without any change to treatment.

Is there any treatment that I can be given to stop my fits if they get very bad?
Yes, there is. Some people with uncontrolled epilepsy are prone to having fits in clusters. Sometimes taking extra medicine in the form of a short-acting drug like a benzodiazepine (see pages 68–70) after the first fit can be effective in preventing the cluster from occurring. If you are unable to take the drug, such as diazepam (Valium), by mouth after you have had a fit, then it can be given to you by injection into the rectum using a special preloaded tube called Stesolid. This contains either 5 mg or 10 mg of diazepam. The usual dose for an adult would be 10 mg or 20 mg. Anyone can

administer the drug this way if they have been shown how to do it and it is quite safe (see diagram on page 44).

Some people find this extremely effective but it's important not to give benzodiazepines very often like this, otherwise the effectiveness wears off and the person can start to get drowsy. This is because the drug begins to build up in the body after repeated doses.

We can cope with our son's fits but the injuries to his head are really terrible. What can we do about them?
Your son probably has tonic or atonic fits (see page 47) in which he falls to the ground abruptly. Although the actual fit may be quite short, injuries to the head and face are common and very distressing. They can also result in facial deformity and scarring.

Some people find that wearing a protective helmet helps prevent the injury and a variety of sports headgear like cycling and ice hockey helmets can be tried. Unfortunately they're often uncomfortable and hot to wear for long periods, and some people understandably hate the idea of wearing one. Commercially available helmets may also not offer the necessary protection when the fit occurs as they often fall off or leave part of the face exposed. Your local hospital appliance department may be able to advise you about getting one specially made for your son.

If you decide against a helmet, or it's not successful in preventing injury, there's not a great deal you can do. The family is then faced with frequent visits to the local casualty department, which may be a great inconvenience. It may be that your local health centre can provide some first aid or teach you what to do if the injury is not too severe.

Our daughter always has more fits when she's constipated. What can we do about it?
Whether constipation really causes people to have more fits is uncertain, because there is no obvious connection between the two.

Quite a lot of parents report that this happens, however. Constipation is very common and can best be dealt with by changing your daughter's diet so she eats more roughage.

Our daughter only has very minor fits but they happen a lot and she wets herself each time. What can we do?
It sounds as if your daughter is having frequent complex absences (see page 47). Wetting or *incontinence* is often a big problem with this type of attack, causing a lot of embarrassment, let alone all the extra washing. Apart from controlling the fits better, there isn't a great deal you can do. Some people with this problem resort to wearing plastic or absorbent pants but usually only as a temporary measure. Going to the toilet very frequently and restricting the amount of fluid drunk may help. But it remains a big handicap to some people.

Our fifteen-year-old son has just started to do better with his fits and he gets on really well with the clinic doctor. But the doctor says he can't see him any more because he's getting too big. What happens now?
This is a problem that faces many young people and one that he should talk to his GP about. A few units have clinics run jointly by doctors seeing children and those seeing adults with epilepsy. This makes the changeover much easier but sadly is only done in a few places. Your GP will probably want to refer your son to see the local neurologist who should be able to offer you the same level of care as provided by the paediatricians. Unfortunately there are only 180 consultant neurologists in the whole country and they are often very busy seeing new patients and dealing with emergencies.

My fits have always been worse around my periods. Will they stop when I reach the menopause?
There isn't a lot of information on this. Certainly the menopause doesn't usually make things any worse but the fits can't be guaranteed to stop either. Removal of the ovaries to produce an early menopause is not recommended.

Should my epilepsy be completely reassessed?
If there are specific questions which still need an answer, then a complete reassessment can be very helpful. It may reveal factors which are making the problem much worse. But merely organizing more tests without a specific objective in mind can be a waste of your time and lead to further disappointment.

There are a number of centres which specialize in helping people with the more severe forms of epilepsy, and their names and addresses can be found in the list below. Your doctor may be able to tell you more about them and the centres themselves will be able to give you more information about how you go about being referred.

What would happen if I went to one of these special centres?
This rather depends on the problems that you are facing. The special centres can reassess the diagnosis and classification of your seizures, review the treatment that you have had and look at any other problems and disabilities that may be present. The assessments are mostly done on a residential basis and the length of stay could be several weeks or even longer if the problems need a lot of sorting out.

NHS epilepsy units and assessment centres

Bootham Park Hospital
Bootham
York YO3 7BY
Tel: 0904 61077
(Medical Director: Dr Pamela Crawford)

Chalfont Centre for Epilepsy
Assessment Unit
Chesham Lane
Chalfont St Peter
Bucks SL9 ORJ

Tel: 02407 3991
(Medical Director: Dr Simon Shorvon)

David Lewis Centre for Epilepsy
Mill Lane
Warford
Nr Alderley Edge
Cheshire SK9 7UD
Tel: 056587 2613
(Consultant: Dr Stephen Brown)

Maudsley Hospital
Epilepsy Unit
Denmark Hill
London SE5 8AZ
Tel: 071-703 6333
(Consultant: Dr Peter Fenwick)

Park Hospital for Children
Old Road
Headington
Oxford OX3 7LQ
Tel: 0865 245651

University of Wales College of Medicine
Epilepsy Unit
Heath Park
Cardiff CF4 4XW
Tel: 0222 747747
(Director: Professor Alan Richens)

For those young people who need a lot of help to become more independent despite continuing to have seizures, the centres also offer training programmes leading to more independent living. Some centres also provide other services such as education, respite care and long-term residential facilities.

If there is no treatment that will stop my fits, is there any point in continuing to see a specialist?

If your epilepsy has not come under full control, it is probably a good idea to continue to see a specialist from time to time. An expert is in a position to advise you about a lot of issues, such as using different combinations of drugs, long-term problems with drugs or even stopping drugs altogether. A specialist is likely to be more aware of new research in epilepsy and new treatments as they become available.

But some people in this situation prefer not to have to go to the hospital clinic for regular visits and your GP can act as your adviser and an effective link, re-referring you to the specialist when the need arises. Some specialists are also happy to allow patients they know to make appointments to be seen if there are any new developments or problems.

Does it matter that I often see a different doctor on each occasion I go to the hospital?

Yes, we think it does matter. But unfortunately the way the NHS is organized means that people with disabilities are often seen by junior doctors in the hospital clinic. As the junior doctors are still in training they change jobs quite frequently and some may not be very knowledgeable about managing complicated cases. You can always ask to see the consultant if you have a particular problem, but it's best to ask for a special appointment to make sure that the consultant can see you on the day that you attend. There are a few units which have special epilepsy clinics where continuity is likely to be better. Nevertheless this is a weakness in our health system. If you find your clinic arrangements unsatisfactory, discuss them with your consultant or your GP.

Being me, making relationships

Our son doesn't seem to be able to make friends of his own age. I think they reject him because of his fits. What can we do?

Certainly seizures can deter some people from making friends, particularly if they are not very knowledgeable about the condition. They may appear not to want to know your son because his fits frighten them and they don't know how to cope. But making friends is also a social skill and it could be that your son lacks some abilities to get on well with other people of his own age group. This may have arisen if he is used to spending a lot of time with you rather than with other young people.

It can be quite difficult for the family to realize how someone they care about comes across to others. Social skills training is often available in adult education and work training units and may be very helpful in this situation.

I really want to live away from home but my parents think that it wouldn't be safe. Can I do it?

It's quite natural to want to live away from your parents once you have grown up. It's also quite natural for your parents to be worried about this. Most people with epilepsy manage well, even if they're still having seizures. Naturally, you need to think carefully about the risks – of accidents at home, travelling and so on – and plan ways of keeping the risks to a minimum. It's probably a good idea to live with other people rather than moving straight away to live on your own. This would give your parents the reassurance that there are people around, if you need help.

The voluntary organizations (see pages 144–5) have some good information on this topic. But if your fits are very frequent, you might benefit from a spell at a special epilepsy centre where you can be taught about caring for yourself.

My daughter wants to be independent so badly but she just doesn't realize how serious her condition is. How can we help her?

This isn't an easy situation. On the one hand you obviously want to support and encourage her but on the other you feel that the severity or frequency of her fits makes living independently quite dangerous.

Epilepsy is unusual in that the people affected may often know very little about the problem other than the fact that they black out occasionally. Being unconscious, they have no first hand knowledge or memory of what actually happens. Some parents, quite understandably, tend to play down the fits by saying, 'You just had one of your turns' or words to that effect.

It's pretty important that adults with epilepsy know as much as possible about their own condition, including what actually happens and what effect this has on other people. You may find it difficult to describe to your daughter exactly what happens but with this information she can then make an informed judgement about the risks that she wants to take.

Where can I find suitable accommodation for my grown-up son who still has fits?

Most local authorities and a lot of housing associations will make special arrangements for people with disabilities, including epilepsy. Sometimes this includes providing some supervision or support, as in a group home.

But before looking for somewhere to live, it's important that your son knows how to look after himself. It can be quite a shock for a young person to try to live without parents around to do everything! Learning how often takes time as it's a question of building up confidence. Local education authorities and epilepsy centres offer training programmes in independent living. The St Katherine's Housing Association based near Croydon provides a range of accommodation with teaching in independent living skills for people with epilepsy. The Association's address is on page 147.

My daughter will never be able to look after herself so I want to find somewhere which will look after her permanently. Where will I find a suitable place?

You may find this difficult for a number of reasons. The days when there were large institutions that would willingly look after people indefinitely are fortunately gone. Unfortunately there are still not enough services on a smaller scale in the community for people with special living needs. Many people remain dependent on their families where this is clearly not in the best interest of either the family or of the disabled person because there is no alternative accommodation with the right level of support.

You may also find that other people have a different view of your daughter's capabilities and they may think that she is capable of more. So many places specialize in rehabilitation work rather than just providing care on a long-term basis.

So perhaps an easier way to look at the situation is to identify what your daughter's present needs are and then to look for an appropriate facility. Your local Social Services department will tell you what's available in your home area and the epilepsy centres can tell you about rehabilitation services and residential care. Their addresses are on pages 144–7. Your local authority will need to be involved in any arrangements as it will be responsible for paying the fees if the place chosen is not run by the authority.

Can I live on my own?

This depends on a number of factors which need careful thought. In general, people whose seizures are at all frequent need to take some extra precautions in the home. A flat may be safer than a house with a lot of stairs, for example. There is a risk while cooking, and the kitchen should be made as safe as possible, with a guard around the cooker. Use pans without protruding handles, so they are less likely to be knocked over if you should fall. You should be very careful about carrying hot dishes around, particularly kettles or pans of boiling water. Microwave ovens are a safer way of heating food than conventional cookers. For obvious reasons, it is better not to have a lot of furniture with sharp corners in the house, although you won't be able to avoid all hazardous objects. Radiators and fires should have a guard. It's also wise to shower rather than take a bath, and you need to have a telephone. You may be able to get some financial help for these aids from your local Social Services department (Social Work department in Scotland).

If you do live alone, making regular contact with your family, friends, neighbours or a social worker will help to reassure them that you're all right.

The list below covers some of the things you can do to make your home environment safer.

Making your house safer

Cookers

- Use a cooker guard
- Turn pan handles to the back of the cooker
- Consider using a microwave
- Do not carry hot dishes about

Fires

- Have good fireguards
- Avoid freestanding heaters

Glass

- Consider having toughened glass fitted in doors if there is a risk of breakage during a seizure

Baths

- Bathe in a shallow bath
- A shower may be safer

- Never use very hot water
- Do not shower or bathe while alone in the house

Pillows

- Consider using a safety pillow, or none at all

Doors to lavatories and bathrooms

- If doors open outwards, the door will not be blocked if you fall behind it

I don't seem to have much interest in sex. Is this because of my epilepsy?
Not everyone has the same level of sex drive and so you shouldn't necessarily think that this is abnormal. Equally there are many possible ways in which the epilepsy may have affected your sexual feelings. Both frequent seizures and the epilepsy drugs can affect the body's hormones although exactly how this affects sexual feelings isn't entirely clear. Mental depression could also be responsible and so could a lack of opportunity for social contact, if you feel inhibited from meeting other people because of your epilepsy. Expert assessment may well help you although there may not be a simple answer to this problem.

I've met someone I want to marry but I'm wondering whether he really wants to live with someone who has fits. Can you advise me?
Any intended partner needs to know a lot about you. It is likely that he knows next to nothing about epilepsy, and what it means to live with it. So he needs to know, in some detail, about your fits and the effect they may have on your life together.

The other aspect to this question concerns your feelings about yourself. Having epilepsy is nothing to be ashamed of, but it seems that you feel unsure about whether the person you wish to marry will be really able to accept you. It is important to discuss these feelings openly before you get married. You may find that an epilepsy group would help you to get in contact with other people who have had these kinds of worry.

I'm still having fits – do you think I could manage a baby?
Many women with epilepsy have had babies and manage them well. It is, of course, better if your fits come under control before you start having a family. But if this seems unlikely to happen, you may want to go ahead anyway.

The main difficulty for mothers with epilepsy is the possibility of accidentally injuring the baby during a seizure. Probably the most practical thing to do is to take advice from other women who have faced this situation. An epilepsy support group would be helpful. Also, a book called *Living with Epilepsy* by Dr David Chadwick and Sue Usiskin deals with this question from first-hand experience.

How can I lower the risk of accidents while I'm looking after my baby?
Apart from the usual precautions in the house (see pages 118–19), there are a few special precautions you should take. Don't bathe the baby on your own, and it's better to change nappies and clothes on the floor. Try to use a push-chair as much as possible rather than carrying the baby, in case you fall. The push-chair can be fitted with a special locking device; advice about this is available from the British Epilepsy Association (see page 144).

It's also a great help to have another person around, especially when the baby is small, so you should take advantage of help which is offered to you by your husband, family, friends and other groups.

Is it safe to breast-feed?
Yes, it is, and your breast milk will certainly be good for your baby. The important points about your drugs are dealt with on page 104. If you are likely to have fits, you'll need to take extra safety precautions. These might include feeding the baby while you are sitting on the floor and only breast-feeding when someone else is there. You could run into problems with having to get up during the night and

losing sleep, so maybe your partner can take this on, giving the baby your breast milk from a bottle. You can express your breast milk directly into the bottle and keep it in the fridge until it is needed.

Family life

Our younger daughter seems to be very sulky and difficult since our son started to have fits. Is this normal and what can we do about it?
Any serious illness in a family member can affect the whole family. It's quite possible that you and your husband have been worried about your son, and perhaps your daughter feels jealous. In caring for your son, you may, inadvertently, have overlooked your daughter's needs. By her behaviour she may be telling you that she, too, wants some special attention.

My wife's so worried by our daughter's fits that she hardly lets her do anything. I don't agree at all, and we have terrible arguments about it. What's the answer?
All parents worry about their children, and some are more protective than others. Deciding how much to worry about a child who has fits is very difficult, as some normal activities do carry greater risk for children with epilepsy. So parents are faced with the problem of taking good care of their child while allowing them to become independent, with the dangers that may bring.

If you and your wife cannot agree, it's likely to be confusing and distressing for all of you, especially your daughter. You may need to get some outside advice. Some parents have found the opportunity to talk to other parents very helpful, and going to an epilepsy support group could be valuable. The voluntary organizations will be able to tell you if there is a group near you (see pages 144–5).

My husband just seems to ignore our eldest boy since he's had fits. Why's he doing this?

It's not only your son who has to come to terms with epilepsy, but everyone in the family. For parents, illness in a child brings up a lot of mixed feelings. Worry and concern are universal, and everyone accepts that. But sometimes more complicated and difficult feelings arise, which are harder to show and speak about.

It may be that your husband is disappointed; he may have had high hopes for your son's future which he now feels, quite wrongly, will not be realized. He may feel guilty or ashamed, or find it difficult to accept that your son is not 'perfect' any more. These feelings are not 'good' or 'bad', but part of the reaction many people have to illness in themselves or a family member. Your husband may need some help. This could come from inside or outside the family and might help him to accept his feelings about what has happened.

Sometimes, when I see my daughter having yet another fit, I wish she wouldn't recover so that she could be free of this terrible problem. Am I the only one who's had this thought?

No, you're not, although not many parents will admit that they have felt as desperate as this. It's good that you are able to look at your feelings about this. It's quite a normal reaction to want to free your child of what you see as a terrible handicap. In some ways epilepsy is often worse for carers than for sufferers as they often know very little about what happens in a fit. You would probably benefit from talking over your feelings with a counsellor.

Since our son started having fits, my wife isn't interested in having sex any more. Is this my fault?

No, it probably isn't anybody's fault, but rather a normal reaction to the stress that epilepsy can bring some families. When one of your own children has such obvious needs, it's often a bit difficult to think of your own, particularly if they are purely for pleasure and involve giving full attention to someone else. Certainly for you to have a good sex life may prove very difficult if you are both worrying about how your son is doing at school, whether he's on the right drugs, or indeed whether he may be having another fit in the bedroom next to yours. It may be that your wife has seen this as a problem as well but you've not been able to talk about it. But it's important to do so.

We feel quite OK about our son's epilepsy and we think he's pretty well adjusted to it too. But his granny just doesn't want to know. She'll never talk about it and says that we shouldn't tell anyone. How can we help her see it our way?

Attitudes to epilepsy, like all disabilities, have changed, and your mother may be reflecting how people reacted when she was younger. Equally she may have personal feelings, even guilt, about your son which she doesn't want to look at. Perhaps she might respond better to someone of her own generation who feels the way you do.

We've been told that our daughter's child mustn't have inoculations because of our son's epilepsy. Is this right?

No, it isn't. You've been told this because it was feared at one time that a baby would be at risk from brain damage if it were immunized against whooping cough and there was a history of epilepsy in the family. Whooping cough is also called *pertussis*. In fact, it has recently been decided that there is no connection between brain damage and whooping cough vaccine. Some doctors nevertheless recommend that whooping cough vaccine should not be given to a child if a first degree relative has a history of fits, that is to say the father, mother, or a brother or a sister. All other immunizations should certainly be given.

Getting on at school

Our son isn't doing very well at school because of his fits. What can be done about this?

This is a serious problem, because it's important that your son gains as much as possible from his schooling, to prepare him for a full life later on. We shouldn't just assume that he's not doing well because of his fits, however. Difficulties at school may have a number of causes, including:

1 Frequent seizures, particularly absence seizures affecting concentration and attention.
2 The effect of anti-epileptic drugs, especially drugs such as phenobarbitone. Drugs for epilepsy can have a number of effects on mental functioning, including poor memory, bad concentration and sleepiness.
3 Damage to the brain, which may be quite minor, and affect only one area – such as arithmetic or reading.
4 Unhappiness due to teasing or bullying.
5 Teachers assuming that he's not as capable as he really is.

You should try to get an idea from his teacher of the exact problem at school, and then discuss this with your son's doctor. The most important thing is not to assume that just because your son has epilepsy he won't do well at school. A full review of the situation, perhaps including an assessment by an educational psychologist, should make it clear how your son's progress at school may be improved.

The kids at school are teasing my son since he had a fit in the playground. What can we do?

There are two aspects to this situation. First, you will need to talk it over with your son. He will need a chance to talk about his feelings and perhaps you will be able to help him understand that people can, sadly, sometimes be unkind to people who happen to be different. If you, and the family, can help him to look at what is happening, it should stop him feeling bad about himself.

Second, you could consider talking to his teacher. If the teacher, and his class-mates, don't know much about epilepsy, it may be an opportunity for some education within the school about what fits are and what it is like for children who have them. The voluntary organizations produce a variety of resource material for teachers and brief details are given in the list below.

British Epilepsy Association
A Guide for Teachers (16 pp A5 booklet)
The Child with Epilepsy (16 pp A5 booklet)
An audiovisual training pack for teachers is in production at the time of writing

Scottish Epilepsy Association
Guidelines for Teachers (booklet)
Training pack on epilepsy for teachers and parents

National Society for Epilepsy
Teachers' training package containing a video and back-up educational material

The teacher says that on some days our son is very alert but on others he hardly takes in anything at all. We've noticed this at home too. What's going on? Is it his drugs?
No, it's probably not his drugs, as the levels of these will be fairly constant from day to day. It could be that he has a lot of activity in his brain that is not actually producing an obvious fit but is nevertheless affecting his ability to think and concentrate. This is called *sub-clinical epileptic activity*. You should ask the teacher for more details and your own observations can be very helpful. For example, when your son is not very well, can you hold a conversation with him and does he talk sensibly? What about his movements? Is he very clumsy? And have you seen anything unusual like flickering of the eyelids and movement of the lips? He may need an EEG at the time this is happening in order to sort out the problem.

A few children, usually with the severe forms of epilepsy, can become vacant and inaccessible for very long periods, even days. An EEG may show persistent epilepsy activity, and the term *absence status* is used to describe this rare condition. It may require an injection into an arm vein to stop it.

Would special schooling be better for my daughter, who has really bad fits?

This rather depends on her educational needs and how these can best be met. Since the 1981 Education Act, there's been a policy that as many children as possible with special educational needs should be educated in ordinary schools. Children with handicaps can also benefit from a full assessment of their abilities and difficulties, leading in some cases to a formal statement or record being prepared. Parents have to be fully involved in this process.

If all those involved decide that some kind of special schooling would help your daughter, this will usually be available at her present school or in one near your home. Occasionally, a special school away from your home area will be suggested and you will need to think this over very carefully as it might mean your daughter being away from home during the term.

There are a few schools that specialize in teaching children with epilepsy and these are listed here. They will be able to give you more information about the facilities that they have. Your Local Authority will have to agree to your daughter attending one of these schools as it will have to pay the fees.

Schools specializing in children with epilepsy

David Lewis School
Mill Lane
Warford
Nr Alderley Edge
Cheshire SK9 7UD

Tel: 056587 2613
(Consultant: Dr Stephen Brown)

St Piers, Lingfield
St Piers Lane
Lingfield
Surrey RH7 6PN
Tel: 0342 832243
(Medical Director: Dr Frank Besag)

St Elizabeth's School
South End
Much Hadham
Hertfordshire SG10 6EW
Tel: 027984 3451

What jobs can our son do when he leaves school?
Your best bet is to get advice as soon as you can from your local
careers service and, if necessary, the specialist careers officers for
people with a disability. Matching your son to a job involves looking at
his abilities and ambitions first and only then asking how the epilepsy
might affect his prospects of getting a job in his chosen field. There
are only a few jobs that are actually barred to a person with a history of
fits but other problems will be found in a wider range of occupations
if the fits are still occurring. Please see page 96 for more details.

*Our son is sixteen, and he won't do anything we tell him – including taking
his tablets. What is the best way to handle him?*
Teenagers are well known for being rebellious and difficult. This is
largely because they are going through the process of developing
their own identity and growing away from the family. So they want to
make their own decisions and not take orders from their parents or
doctors. At the same time, they want to be just like their friends, and
often resent anything which makes them seem different. Taking
tablets can be a very unwelcome reminder that they are not quite the
same as their friends.

It's wise not to make tablets too much of a battleground. Giving your son as much control as possible for his tablets and medical care is a good idea, while stating your views firmly and clearly. If possible, try to deflect struggles on to other areas. His rebellion will probably not last too long.

Our daughter was a happy child, but she is fourteen now and seems miserable all the time. Is it her epilepsy?
It may be. Teenagers have a lot to cope with – changing relationships, sexuality, school pressures – and your daughter may be unhappy about any of these things. She's also at a stage where she's moving out into the world from the security of her family. Her fits, and whether people will accept her, may be an added worry for her.

It's also worth considering whether her medicine is affecting her mood, and you should discuss this with her doctor. If her unhappiness seems to be long-lasting and severe, she may benefit from professional counselling or treatment.

My daughter's fits are very bad sometimes and we are getting older. We are worried about the future. Where can we get help?
Parents very naturally fear for the future and often think that there are no suitable facilities which will provide the sort of care that they do. They are probably right. But quite often even people severely disabled by fits can become much more independent than you might think. But it takes time and a lot of courage. Going to an epilepsy support group might give you the chance to meet other parents in the same situation.

Your Local Authority Social Services department (Social Work department in Scotland) will be able to tell you what facilities exist where you live, and the voluntary organizations may be able to tell you about other services. You can then think about what sort of help your daughter needs now and in the future. But you need to give everyone plenty of time because your daughter will have her own wishes and needs and it may be difficult to find exactly the right set-up for her. Special facilities in the community are being developed partly as a result of the Disabled Persons (Representations) Act of 1986.

When seizures are not the only problem

You say that people with epilepsy are just the same as other people, apart from when they're having a fit. But there's a boy in our village who has fits and he doesn't seem at all normal to me. Can you explain this?
It isn't very easy to explain this! Having epilepsy only causes someone to be liable to have fits. It does not make them physically disabled or mentally handicapped. So unless they're actually having a fit at the time, you can't see any outward signs of the epilepsy. The vast majority of people with epilepsy are therefore 'normal' in the sense that they don't have any other handicaps. What you are probably seeing in this boy is not his epilepsy but rather the outward signs of brain damage. This brain damage may itself be the cause of his epilepsy.

People often only know that someone has epilepsy when there are obvious handicaps as well. This tends to mean that the general public gets the wrong idea about epilepsy. For example, people with epilepsy who are successful in business or their social life often keep quiet about it. Although we would probably do the same thing in their place, this approach does nothing to counteract the stereotype that many have about epilepsy. This part of the chapter concentrates on the other handicaps that can sometimes accompany having epilepsy.

Our daughter is also mentally handicapped. Should her epilepsy be treated in the same way as everyone else's?
In general the answer is, yes. People with a mental handicap need all the expertise and facilities that other people with epilepsy get. Epilepsy is a common problem when mental handicap is present but quite often the fits are easy to control.

Assessing and treating seizures in people with a mental handicap can be more difficult for a number of reasons. Your daughter may, for example, find it hard to let you know how she feels and how her drugs are affecting her. Teaching her to look after her own medicine may be a challenge, needing extra time and effort.

Drug dosages should be kept as low as possible: sometimes inappropriate drug treatment may result from not classifying her fits properly. Unusual behaviour patterns can easily be mistaken for seizures. Although doctors who look after people with mental handicap often know a lot about epilepsy, there are very few units which specialize in this double disability. Even if your daughter's seizures remain a problem, a lot can be done to teach her, your whole family and her other professional supporters about managing the problems in the best way.

We've been told that our son has the Lennox-Gastaut syndrome. *What can we expect to happen to him?*
Some forms of severe epilepsy follow particular patterns and these may be grouped together in what is called a *syndrome*. This one was described by two famous neurologists and it was named after them. As you will already have found out, epilepsy is not the only problem in this syndrome and a varying degree of mental handicap is also usually present.

People with the Lennox-Gastaut syndrome often have more than one type of fit; usually a combination of complex absences, atonic, tonic and tonic-clonic seizures. These often do not respond well to drugs. Falls with injury to the head are common. So the outlook is not very good and people with this problem often need special care and their families need extra support.

Our son can't do the things he used to be able to do. Is it the drugs that are affecting him?
It may be, particularly if he is on a lot of medicine. Reviewing his treatment may be worthwhile but unfortunately reducing his

dosage could also lead to more attacks.

There are a number of other causes of failing ability. As children get older we expect more of them and so what you see as deterioration may just be that your son is failing to keep up with other children of his own age. But it's worth trying to identify what exactly he can't do now that he used to be able to do. This would be valuable information for an expert who may need to assess what is going on. Frequent seizures, particularly if he also injures his head a lot, can themselves lead to brain damage. If no treatable cause can be found, then an expert assessment from a clinical psychologist may help you to identify your son's main strengths and weaknesses so that you can all help him make the best use of his abilities.

Our son has also become very unsteady on his feet and his speech is slurred. What's happening to him?
It sounds as if the back part of the brain, known as the brain stem and the cerebellum has been damaged. This is the part of the brain that controls balance and our ability to say words clearly. The difficulty with balance is known technically as *ataxia* and the slurring of speech is called *dysarthria*.

There are two main causes of this problem. The first is too high a level of epilepsy drugs and the second is damage caused by repeated head injuries. It may be necessary to measure the levels of the drugs in his blood and if these are very high, a reduction in dose may help. If this is not the cause, then a CT scan may show up the damage. Unfortunately, if this is present, there is no specific treatment available which will reverse the damage. Physiotherapy and speech therapy may help, however.

I have such a terrible memory. Why is this and what can I do about it?
We don't fully understand why some people with epilepsy have this problem. It may be partly due to the fits interrupting the normal ways in which the brain makes us remember things. It may also be partly due to the drugs. Unfortunately, it isn't an easy problem to

tackle. But keeping a diary and using various tricks such as rhymes and memory 'cues' may help. The book by Sander and Thompson deals with this problem in more depth. Please see the end of the chapter for details.

My wife's fits are not too bad but she keeps having these bouts of depression. What's causing it?
It's difficult to answer this precisely without knowing more about your wife. Depression is a common experience in our society, and it does occur more commonly in people with epilepsy. Research into this area has indicated that people with epilepsy may become depressed for a number of reasons. First, some of the anti-epileptic drugs can cause depression. Phenobarbitone is particularly bad for this. Second, coping with a disorder like epilepsy can be depressing for some people. Loss of self-esteem, restricted activities and employment problems are the kinds of experience that may promote depression. It has also been thought that depression may be directly related to the changes in the brain that occur in epilepsy – but this idea has not been proven.

Whatever the cause of your wife's depression, she should consult her doctor, and perhaps she might consider seeing a psychiatrist for expert advice on the problem and possible treatment.

Can my wife's depression be treated despite her fits?
Yes, it can be, but the most appropriate form of treatment will depend on the severity of her symptoms and their cause. Your wife may require counselling or some form of psychotherapy. Drug treatment may also be indicated in some circumstances and usually these can be used safely in people with epilepsy although some doctors are cautious about using drugs for depression (anti-depressants) because they can upset the control of fits. It's important not just to put up with the depression thinking that it's just part of having epilepsy.

My husband gets so violent sometimes that I think he might hurt someone.
I think that it's his fits that make him this way. Am I right?
Violent behaviour directed at someone else is very rarely caused by
fits. However, the confused behaviour after a fit can be mistaken for
deliberate aggression by people who don't know about the epilepsy,
particularly if attempts are made to restrain the person who has had
the fit. We discuss how to deal with fits on pages 26-8.

Unfortunately people with epilepsy can be violent for all the same
reasons that make other people violent, such as the way they have
been brought up, personality problems, alcohol and illegal drugs.
But as your husband has epilepsy there could be other causes, such
as brain damage or his epilepsy treatment. In a small number of
people epilepsy drugs can increase a tendency towards violent
behaviour. You really need to get an expert opinion.

Is it true that the law considers someone with epilepsy to be insane if they do
something wrong during a fit?
Unfortunately, as the law stands in the UK at present, this is the
case. If a person commits an offence in the confused state after a fit
(for example injuring a bystander), then a plea of 'not guilty because
of epilepsy' is the same as 'not guilty because of insanity'. The law
does not distinguish between the mental state of a person after a fit
and the mental state of someone suffering from a mental illness. If a
person enters 'epilepsy' as a plea, then they run the risk of being
sent to a secure hospital, such as Broadmoor. Epilepsy experts have
pointed out the injustice in this situation and not all courts will
interpret the law in this way. Expert legal and medical advice is
essential if a person with epilepsy is accused of an offence alleged to
have been committed as a result of a fit.

My mother started having fits following a stroke. Her right arm shakes in a
fit and it seems very weak for ages afterwards. Is this normal?
Epilepsy is quite common in older people and it is nearly always due
to some damage to the brain such as can occur during a stroke.

Other causes include brain tumours and simple shrinkage of the brain due to old age (also called *atrophy*). As a result older people quite often have partial seizures (see pages 49–51) and they may or may not go unconscious in a fit.

Your mother's fits sound like partial seizures affecting the left side of her brain towards the front in the area called the *motor cortex*. That part of her brain hasn't recovered fully after the stroke. When she has a fit it is quite usual, particularly if the fit lasts a long time, for the arm to be much weaker for several hours afterwards or even longer. If the weakness persists or seems to be getting worse then you should let her doctor know.

Keeping active

I haven't been able to get a job since leaving school because of my fits. Who can help me?
Getting a job can be difficult for anyone, and having active epilepsy is quite likely to make it more difficult for you. However, lots of people still having seizures do get paid jobs and some who don't do voluntary work instead. You may already have received careers advice while at school from your careers teacher and your careers officer. Your next step is to get further advice from a Careers Officer at your local Careers Office. You may be recommended to see the specialist careers officer who will liaise with the Disablement Resettlement Officer (DRO for short).

The DRO will want some details about your epilepsy and the way your fits might affect your work abilities. Sometimes further work assessment or training at one of the special colleges for young people with disabilities is suggested or you may be given the opportunity to join one of the government schemes for young people.

Perhaps you've not been successful at job interviews because you don't go about selling yourself to an employer very well – the DRO can help you by suggesting you attend a Job Club where you can get help with interview technique. If the DRO finds an employer who is willing to employ you but who still has doubts about employing someone with epilepsy, the Job Introduction Scheme might be used. You could also ask one of the voluntary organizations to talk to the employer and give guidance about employing someone with epilepsy.

Should I register as disabled? Will this help me get a job?
It might do. If the DRO rates your disability as being fairly severe, you might be encouraged to register as disabled for the purposes of employment. Quite a lot of people are worried about doing this, thinking that it labels them as different. It's true that registering is not a passport to getting a job but it does allow the DRO to suggest that you are employed under the Quota Scheme, which requires employers with more than twenty employees to have at least 3 per cent of them as registered disabled people.

You could also be employed under the Sheltered Employment Programme either in a sheltered workshop or Remploy factory or on the Sheltered Placement Scheme. About 20,000 people in the UK are employed under this programme.

I want to play sport and swim but I often find it difficult to find anywhere that will accept me. What can I do about it?
Most local authority-run swimming pools and recreation centres make special provision for people with disabilities. They may want to restrict your attendance to specific times when people with disabilities are given priority and you might find this annoying, preferring to use the facilities with other members of the general public. Privately run sports facilities may well not be so welcoming and you would do well to approach them informally first. If you don't get the welcome that you hope for, you could try to turn the meeting into an educational experience for them!

Whenever you go swimming, you should always let the attendant know about your epilepsy and the way in which it might affect you should a fit occur. You could well get a hostile reception if a fit occurred and no one was prepared for it. Some people with epilepsy adopt the 'buddy' system. Under this scheme they take a friend along with them, whom they know well and who knows exactly what to do if a fit occurs.

Is it safe for me to travel abroad?
Yes, there's no reason at all why you shouldn't travel abroad, but you've got a lot to think about. You may, for example, have some difficulty getting full insurance cover and so you should give your travel agent plenty of notice and read the small print carefully as existing health problems may be excluded from some policies. The British Epilepsy Association can arrange a travel insurance policy for you.

If you are travelling to an EC country you need to obtain form E111 before you go, so that if you need any medical treatment while abroad, you can claim all or part of the expenses under the NHS.

Flying should not present a problem but it's worth letting the airline know in advance about your fits and how they could affect you. If fits are at all likely, you might decide that it is better to have someone with you who knows you. Other forms of transport abroad should not be a problem.

You will also have to remember to take enough medicine with you for your journey and for the time you will be abroad (see page 40). Some people with epilepsy who travel frequently recommend that you keep your medicine with you and don't pack it in your main luggage which can always go astray. If you are crossing time zones, you should try to keep your dosages as regular as you can but you may have to make some adjustments over a number of days. Very long flights during which your normal sleep pattern might be upset could be hazardous if your attacks have been brought on by lack of sleep in the past.

If you are going to a country where you need inoculations, you will need to discuss having these with your doctor in plenty of time. You can have all the immunizations quite safely.

What social security benefits am I entitled to?
The benefits you can get depend on the way that your epilepsy has
affected your ability to earn a living and your present financial
circumstances. There are no benefits specifically for having epilepsy and the arrangements change very frequently. The best
people to advise you are your local Social Security benefits office,
your social worker or other adviser, and the voluntary organizations (see pages 144–5).

Helping others

What is a self-help group and would it help me?
The self-help movement is now well established in this country as
in many others. It's based on the principle that people who share a
condition have a lot to offer each other because of their different
experiences of living with the condition. There are now quite a
few groups up and down the country made up of people with
epilepsy and their families. Professionals may play a part as well in
some groups.

   Groups vary tremendously in what they do. All will offer support to people facing the problems of epilepsy for the first time.
Some are also involved in public education and others are active
fund-raisers. Whether such a group will help you largely depends
on your needs and what you feel able to contribute. The voluntary
organizations can give you more information. Their addresses are
on pages 144–5.

What can I do to help other people like me?
You can do a lot. Even people who seem to have the most severe
problems often say that there are people worse off than themselves. So you're bound to have something to offer.

   One way to come to a decision on how you can help is to look at
what you're good at. You may have some particular skill or experience from which other people or organizations could benefit. All

the voluntary organizations need volunteer help, often for fund-raising or other practical jobs. If you like talking to others you might take up some educational work, and the British Epilepsy Association runs courses for speakers. One of the most valuable contributions you can make is to share your experiences with others facing the problems for the first time, and the local epilepsy support groups would welcome your participation. Last, but sadly by no means least, the epilepsy movement as a whole badly needs funds for the whole range of its activities from scientific research to providing holidays and respite care.

For more information about:

Travel

A Traveller's Handbook for Persons with Epilepsy
International Bureau for Epilepsy
PO Box 21, 2100 AA Heemstede
Holland

Living with seizures

Living with Epilepsy by David Chadwick and Sue Usiskin (Macdonald Optima, 1991) (paperback for patients)

Psychology and memory

Chapter 6 in *Epilepsy: a practical guide to coping* by L. Sander and P. Thompson (Crowood Health Guides) (paperback for patients).

10   Progress now

In the 100 years since the first epilepsy institutions were opened, and in the forty years since the British Epilepsy Association was founded, there has been tremendous progress in our understanding of epilepsy and its consequences.

But for people facing problems today, it's often difficult to see that progress is still going on. The process is so slow that it hardly seems to be there at all. So in this short chapter we look at some of the areas where improvements may be won in the next few years. At the end of this section you will find the addresses of the main epilepsy organizations.

Will there ever be a cure for epilepsy?
Maybe there will be one day. Finding a cure depends on dis-covering what exactly goes wrong in the brain when people start to have fits. Almost certainly there's more than one cause and we need to look at people's genetic make-up as well as the chemistry in their brains. Once we know in more detail what leads people to start having fits, then it will be easier to find a solution to the problem. But this means more research.

What research is going on?
There's a lot of research going on worldwide. A great deal is to do with finding better drugs for epilepsy and this is carried out by the various drug companies. Ten years ago, there were hardly any new drugs being developed and now there are a lot. But not many of

these will make the grade as they will be found either not to work well enough or to cause too many side-effects.

One new drug, vigabatrin (Sabril) was launched in 1989 in the UK and this was the first drug to be specifically designed to treat epilepsy. The other drugs that we use had all been found by chance through screening programmes. Other new drugs may reach the market soon and there has been a lot of work in the UK on two, one called lamotrigine (Lamictal) and the other gabapentin.

Is all the research about new drugs?

No it isn't, although the amount spent in looking for new drugs is huge compared to other kinds of research. Drug companies have a commercial reason for looking for new drugs, whereas other kinds of research have to rely on grants either from Government or, increasingly, from charities. But research into other areas does go on in a number of centres in the UK and some of them are listed on pages 147–8. Main areas of activity at the moment include the basic processes of epilepsy, the best way to withdraw drugs, looking at epilepsy in the general populations of different countries and better ways of assessing people for epilepsy surgery.

How can I help with research?

Some people are asked by their doctors to take part in research projects. Trials of new drugs are considered on page 108. But there are many other kinds of research, some of which only involve you in filling in a questionnaire. The main epilepsy research groups can give you more details and their addresses are on pages 147–8. The one way you could certainly help is by raising money for research. This isn't easy and the amounts needed are very large. But everything helps.

I've heard that there is a new Charter for people with epilepsy. What is it exactly?

The Charter was launched by the British Epilepsy Association (BEA)

The Charter for People with Epilepsy

British Epilepsy Association believes that people with epilepsy:

Are INDIVIDUALS and should be respected and
treated as such

Should be offered education and training opportunities in
the community to suit their needs and abilities

Are entitled to employment policies and procedures based
on their skills, experience and qualifications

Sometimes have particular needs which should be met by a
system of disability benefits and allowances

Deserve quality medical care from practitioners who
understand epilepsy, on a free and accessible basis

Have the right to information to help them choose whether
or not to undergo any treatment offered.

SHOULD BE ABLE TO SAY 'I HAVE EPILEPSY'
WITHOUT BEING REJECTED OR LABELLED BY
OTHERS

---

in September 1990 in a presentation ceremony to its patron, the Duchess of Kent. It contains seven statements summarizing the needs of people with epilepsy (see page 141).

The Association is looking for widespread support for the Charter which is being sent to employers, government, other decision-makers and people with influence everywhere. You can help promote the Charter by signing your name to it. For more details contact the BEA. Its address is on page 144.

Will there ever be a Bill of Rights for people with epilepsy?
It's rather unlikely, as we're not a country that has rights for its citizens spelt out in laws. For a long time there has been support for anti-discrimination laws for all people with disabilities, much as there are for racial minorities. Successive UK governments have not wanted to go down this road, but things could change. The Americans with Disabilities Act was signed by the President of the United States in July 1990 despite a lot of official opposition at the start of the campaign. The Epilepsy Foundation of America, the USA's national organization for people with epilepsy, played a big part in lobbying the US Congress to get support. Getting new laws passed needs a lot of co-ordinated effort by everyone and a lot of money.

How much money is needed to help the epilepsy movement?
It's all a question of investment. The more that is spent now, the less epilepsy should cost in future in terms of treatment, special services and missed opportunities. The amount that is actually spent on helping people with epilepsy by Government and local authorities is not known, but the amounts received as donations by all the UK voluntary organizations put together is less than £1 million a year. This is a much smaller sum than many of the medical charities attract.

An alternative way of looking at the problem would be to ask how much could be raised and what progress could be achieved with this money. Some simple calculations may help. There are 300,000 people with epilepsy in the UK. If each of these people gave £1 per year, the amount raised would be £300,000. If each of these people gave £1 every month the amount raised would be £3.6 million, or three times what the voluntary organizations receive now.

It is said that every person with a disability knows at least ten other people who act as supporters in some way. If each of these people gave £1 per month to the epilepsy movement, you would raise £36 million every year. And so on.

Now, of course it isn't only people with epilepsy and their supporters who should be encouraged to give. And families with epilepsy are often faced with higher than usual costs. But the same is true of other disability groups where the sums raised are much greater than for epilepsy.

Useful addresses

Addresses for NHS epilepsy units and assessment centres are listed on pages 112–13, and for schools specializing in children with epilepsy on pages 126–7.

National epilepsy organizations in the UK and Ireland

British Epilepsy Association
40 Hanover Square
Leeds LS3 1BE
(Chief Executive: Terry O'Leary)
Tel: 0532 439393

> **National Information Centre Helpline** 0345 089599 (calls charged at local rates)

> **BEA Southern Office**
> 72A London Street
> Reading
> Berks. RG1 4SJ
> Tel: 0734 591843

> **BEA Northern Ireland Office**
> The Old Postgraduate Medical Centre
> Belfast City Hospital
> Lisburn Road
> Belfast BT9 7AB
> Tel: 0232 248414

Epilepsy Association of Scotland
48 Govan Road
Glasgow G51 1JL
Tel: 041 427 4911
(Executive director: John Craig)

Irish Epilepsy Association
249 Crumlin Road
Dublin 12
Tel: 1 557500
(Chief Executive: Richard Holmes)

National Society for Epilepsy
Chesham Lane
Chalfont St Peter
Bucks. SL9 0RJ
Tel: 02407 3991
(Chief Executive: David Eking)

Wales Epilepsy Association
Y Pant Teg
Brynteg
Dolgellau
Gwynedd LL40 1RP
(Chairman: J. Roberts)

There may be other local organizations in your area. You can get
more information from your local phone book, the Citizens Advice
Bureau or the national epilepsy organizations.

Centres offering rehabilitation and residential care

Chalfont Centre for Epilepsy
Chesham Lane
Chalfont St Peter
Bucks. SL9 0RJ
Tel: 02407 3991

Croydon Epilepsy Society
8a Ledbury Road
Croydon CR0 1EP
Tel: 081-760 0756

David Lewis Centre for Epilepsy
Mill Lane
Warford
Nr Alderley Edge
Cheshire SK9 7UD
Tel: 0565 872613

Epilepsy Centre
Quarrier's Home
Bridge of Weir
Renfrewshire PA11 3SA
Tel: 0505 612224
(Consultant physician: Dr Jane Gray)

Meath Home
Westbrook Road
Godalming
Surrey GU7 2QJ
Tel: 0483 415095

St Elizabeth's
South End
Much Hadham
Herts. SG10 6EW
Tel: 027984 3451

St Katherine's Housing Association
Ambassador House
Brigstock Road
Thornton Heath
Surrey CR7 7XF
Tel: 081-684 3902

UK epilepsy research organizations

British Epilepsy Research Foundation
40 Hanover Square
Leeds LS3 1BE
Tel: 0532 439393
(Secretary: Terry O'Leary)

Institute of Neurology, National Hospital and National Society for Epilepsy Research Group (INSEG)
Institute of Neurology
Queen Square
London WC1N 3BG
Tel: 071-837 3611/02407 3991
(Director: Dr Simon Shorvon)

University of Wales College of Medicine
Epilepsy Unit
Heath Park
Cardiff CF4 4XW
Tel: 0222 747747
(Director: Professor Alan Richens)

West of Scotland Epilepsy Research Group
Department of Medicine and Therapeutics
Gardiner Institute
Western Infirmary
Glasgow G I I 6NT
Tel: 041 339 8822
(Chairman: Dr Martin Brodie)

International organizations

Epilepsy Foundation of America
4351 Garden City Drive
Landover
Maryland 20785
USA
Tel: 010 1 301 459 3700

International Bureau for Epilepsy (IBE)
(An international organization for people with epilepsy and their supporters)

PO Box 21
2100 AA Heemstede
Holland
Tel: 010 31 23 339060
Commissions on:
   – audio-visual education
   – employment
   – public education
   – self-help
   – travel

The British chapter of the IBE is the British Epilepsy Association

International Epilepsy News
Editors: Richard Masland and Hanneke de Boer
(Address as for IBE)

International League against Epilepsy (ILAE)

(An organization for doctors and other professionals)
Secretary General: Dr Roger Porter
Department of Health and Human Services
National Institute of Health
Building 31
Bethesda
Maryland 20892
USA
Commissions on:
- anti-epileptic drugs
- driving licences (with IBE)
- developing countries (with IBE)
- education
- pregnancy

ILAE British branch secretary: Dr Simon Shorvon, Institute of
Neurology, Queen Square, London WC1N 3BG

Other addresses

Driving licences
The Medical Advisor
Medical Advisory Branch
Department of Transport
Oldway Centre
Orchard Street
Swansea SA1 1ZZ
Tel: 0792 304482

Personal safety aids
Medic-Alert
17 Bridge Wharf
156 Caledonian Road
London N1 9UU
Tel: 071-833 3034

SOS Talisman
Talman Ltd
21 Grays Corner
Ley Street
Ilford
Essex IG2 7RQ
Tel: 081-554 5579

Employment
Employment Medical Advisory Service, see under Health and
Safety Executive in your local phone book

Disablement Resettlement Officer (DRO), contact your local Job
Centre

Index

TV, *see* television

University of Wales, College of
  Medicine, 113, 147
unsteadiness (side-effect), 57, 62, 64,
  131

Valium, *see* diazepam
vigabatrin (drug), 34–5, 55, 140
  need for blood tests, 58
  side-effects of, 57, 60
violence, 133
vision, blurred (side-effect), 64
vitamins, 60
volunteering, 137–8
vomiting (side-effect), 64, 66, 68

Wales Epilepsy Association, 145

for other Welsh organizations, *see*
  University of Wales
warnings
  auras, 3, 31, 51–2, 93, 101
  before partial seizures, 49
  before seizures, 51–2
weight gain (side-effect), 66
West of Scotland Epilepsy Research
  Group, 148
wetting (incontinence), and fits, 111
women, incidence of epilepsy in, 44
work, *see* employment
worsening, of condition, 25, 109, 130–1

yoga, 90

Zarontin, *see* ethosuximide

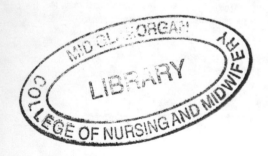

A Selection of
Faber Health Titles

Understanding Your Child
A Parent's Guide to Child Psychology

RICHARD WOOLFSON

All parents are interested in their child's emotional and psychological development. Anxiety can often arise from simple misunderstandings of the child's changing emotional needs and behaviour.

Understanding Your Child is written by a child psychologist and combines practical advice to parents with an outline of the theories underlying the understanding of child development and behaviour. The book starts with a brief explanation of these theories and this is followed by chapters on specific subjects. As well as general topics such as language development and birth order, the book deals with problem areas like aggression, shyness and discipline. Finally there is a 'Development Checklist' to show the stages that children pass through between 0 and 5 years.

A fascinating book for all parents who really want to understand their child.

Faber Paperback   192pp
ISBN 0 571 15382 8   £4.99

The Health Care Consumer Guide

ROBERT GANN

How do you change your doctor? Where do you go for
family planning advice? When do you have to pay for dental
treatment? Which are the best books on everything from
AIDS to sickle cell disease? Can you refuse treatment?
How do you complain about your doctor? How do you get
on the shortest waiting list? Can you have a home birth on
the NHS? Are you covered for health care when you go
abroad?

The answers to all these questions and much, much
more are given in *The Health Care Consumer Guide*.

There are details of your rights as a patient, which
agencies do what, where to go for more information and
what to do when things go wrong. All aspects of health care
are covered. This is a mine of invaluable information for
everyone involved in health care as a consumer or provider.
Robert Gann is a Health Information Manager for Wessex
Health Authority.

Faber Paperback   352pp
ISBN 0 571 14298 2   £7.99

The Epilepsy Reference Book
New Edition

JOLYON OXLEY and JAY SMITH

This is the main information source on epilepsy for
patients, their families, GPs and other health workers. The
diagnosis of epilepsy can have a devastating effect on
people's lives. There is a desperate need for information
on the subject. The new edition of this standard book
covers all aspects of the condition. Details of diagnosis and
medication are followed by information on the incidence
and possible causes of epilepsy. Later chapters deal with
long-term questions related to employment rights, travel,
adjustment, diet, drugs, pregnancy, etc.

As well as helping patients to take more interest in their
condition and form fruitful working partnerships with their
doctors, the book provides information for the numerous
other professionals – nurses, social workers, voluntary
workers – who work with epileptic clients.

Faber Paperback   128pp
ISBN 0 571 16253 3   £4.99

Your Child's Health

IVAN BLUMENTHAL

Dr Ivan Blumenthal is a children's specialist
(paediatrician) trained in the UK and USA: in this book he
presents a comprehensive overview and guide for parents
to the health and environmental hazards facing young
children.

Ranging from problems in growth, behaviour and
learning to the management of classic childhood diseases,
the author has adopted an unpatronizing, matter-of-fact,
yet reassuring tone. Serious conditions such as diabetes,
spina bifida, Down's syndrome, etc. are lucidly explained
and management regimens fully described. Surprising
facts emerge in the discussion about asthma and related
allergies.

Much of the book is in the form of questions that
parents are most likely to ask; and the answers describe
and explain procedures including hospital ones, in a way
that dispels doubts and fears.

A useful list of support groups, in the UK and USA, is
included. So too are further reading lists for both a lay
readership and a professional one.

This book will be valuable not only to parents, but to all
who have the care of children as their concern, such as
teachers, health visitors, nurses, counsellors, social
workers, GPs and others.

Faber Paperback   400pp
ISBN 0 571 14707 0   £6.95

Everywoman

A Gynaecological Guide for Life

DEREK LLEWELLYN-JONES

Everywoman is one of the most successful books ever published on women's health. It has sold nearly two million copies since it was first published in 1971 and has contributed to the awareness which women now have of their bodies and their health needs.

This fifth edition is an updating and revision with new illustrations throughout. There is new material on the AIDS virus and other sexually transmitted diseases which have become more common, early detection of breast cancer, osteoporosis, new pregnancy tests and dietary advice. The sections on complications in pregnancy and tests carried out in pregnancy have been completely revised.

Everywoman has helped millions of women to learn more about themselves. It will continue to do so in this new edition.

Hard covers   416pp
ISBN 0 571 15436 0   £9.99

Faber Paperback   416pp
ISBN 0 571 15321 6   £4.99